Understanding Rheumatoid Arthritis

Rheumatoid arthritis is a major cause of disability affecting about 1 per cent of the population. Although much effort has been expended on research into the causes and treatment of RA, little progress has been made in finding a cure. The focus of treatment in RA is on reducing the disabling consequences of disease and controlling the symptoms.

Understanding Rheumatoid Arthritis examines the nature of RA and its treatment, individuals' experience of RA and its symptoms of pain and stiffness. The impact of RA on quality of life is presented as well as the role of health care professionals and encounters with the doctor, all of which influence the individual's behaviour towards their RA. For instance, some sufferers appear to adapt successfully to their RA while others appear to have difficulty. This book explores the psychological and social aspects of RA in order to contribute to the development of a broad based understanding of RA.

Understanding Rheumatoid Arthritis will be invaluable to all health professionals involved in its treatment and/or interested in chronic illness. It will also be useful to those who suffer from rheumatoid arthritis, their families and carers.

Stanton Newman is Professor of Health Psychology at University College Medical School, University of London; **Ray Fitzpatrick** is a Fellow at Nuffield College and University Lecturer in the Department of Public Health and Primary Care, University of Oxford; **Tracey A. Revenson** is Associate Professor of Psychology at the Graduate School and University Center, City University, New York; **Suzanne Skevington** is Senior Lecturer in Psychology at the School of Social Sciences, University of Bath; **Gareth Williams** is Reader in Sociology of Health and Illness at the Institute of Social Research, University of Salford.

Understanding Rheumatoid Arthritis

Stanton Newman, Ray Fitzpatrick, Tracey A. Revenson, Suzanne Skevington and Gareth Williams

ROUTLEDGE
London and New York

First published 1996
by Routledge
11 New Fetter Lane, London EC4P 4EE

Simultaneously published in the USA and Canada
by Routledge
29 West 35th Street, New York, NY 10001

Typeset in Times by
Florencetype Ltd, Stoodleigh, Devon
Printed and bound in Great Britain by
Clays Ltd, St Ives plc

British Library Cataloguing in Publication Data
A catalogue record for this book is available from the British Library.

Library of Congress Cataloguing in Publication Data
A catalogue record for this book has been requested

ISBN 0–415–10540–4
ISBN 0–415–10541–2 (pbk)

We would like to dedicate this book to all those who confront arthritis and to our colleague Rosemarie Archer who studied these issues with us.

Contents

Tables

Acknowledgements

Ideas for a book come from a variety of sources and we have all been fortunate to have the opportunity to meet and discuss issues on the psychological and social aspects of arthritis. These were facilitated by a Collaborative Senior International Fellowship from the Fogarty International Center of the US National Institute of Health (Grant no. 1 FOG TWO1663) to Tracey Revenson and Stanton Newman. In addition Tracey Revenson was supported by a grant from the New York chapter of the Arthritis Foundation (Fisher Foundation Bequest).

In addition we have been assisted by both our colleagues who have commented on chapters and our collaborators in the studies reported in this volume. Our sincere thanks to Rosemarie Archer, Michael Bury, Barbara Felton, Heather Fields, Allan Gibofsky, Crispin Jenkinson, Ana Abraido-Lanza, Susan Lonsdale, Deborah Majerovitz, Alastair Mowat, Edward Seidman, Kathleen Schiaffino, Michael Shipley. We would also like to thank Sue Garratt for manipulating the text, Sabrina Duncan and Gail Meacham for help with literature searches and Liz Wake for assisting with proofreading.

Acknowledgements

Acronyms

AIMS	Arthritic Impact Measurement Scales
BDI	Beck Depression Inventory
CES-D	Centre for Epidemiological Studies – Depression
CNS	central nervous system
CSQ	Coping Strategies Questionnaire
DIS	Diagnostic Interview Schedule
DMARD	Disease modifying and reducing drugs
EA	experimentally induced arthritis
EMG	electromyograph
ESR	erythrocyte sedimentation rate
FSI	Functional Status Index
GHQ	General Health Questionnaire
HAD	Hospital Anxiety and Depression Scale
HAQ	Health Assessment Questionnaire
MPQ	McGill Pain Questionnaire
NHP	Nottingham Health Profile
NSAIDs	non-steroidal anti-inflammatory drugs
OA	osteoarthritis
PDI	Pain Disability Index
QoL	quality of life
QWB	Quality of Well-being
RA	rheumatoid arthritis
RADAR	Rapid Assessment of Disease Activity in Rheumatology
SAARD	slow-acting antirheumatic drugs
SEIQoL	Schedule for the Evaluation of Individual Quality of Life
SIP	Sickness Impact Profile

SNS	sympathetic nervous system
VAPRS	Visual Analogue of Pain Relief Scale
VAS	Visual Analogue Scale
VMPMI	Vanderbilt Multidimensional Pain Management Inventory
VPCI	Vanderbilt Pain Coping Inventory
WOC	Ways of Coping

Chapter 1

Introduction

Rheumatoid arthritis (RA) is a major cause of disability affecting about 1 per cent of the population. This disability results from changes in the anatomy and functioning of the joints. The main symptoms individuals with RA report are pain, stiffness, joint swelling and fatigue. The course of RA, in its most common form, consists of a series of flares where the disease worsens, followed by periods of remission. In most cases there is a steady trend towards increasing disability over the lifetime of the disease. Among a small proportion of people the disease takes on a more advanced form where the move towards severe disablement is rapid.

Although much effort has been expended on research into the causes of RA little progress has been made. The search for a cure continues, but in this sphere as well, progress has been limited. The focus of treatment in RA is on reducing the disabling consequences of disease and controlling the symptoms. The main thrust of treatment has been pharmacological where the development and use of non-steroidal anti-inflammatory drugs (NSAIDs) for controlling inflammation and stiffness are widely used. Analgesics are most often used to control pain. Where NSAIDs are not successful alternative drugs are available and in use. Surgery for joint replacement is performed where the damage to the joint is irreversible and severely disabling. A variety of non-medical interventions are also used by individuals who have RA. Physiotherapy is the most popular, frequently used as an adjunct to medical treatments. Others include a variety of interventions for pain control, weight-loss regimes and self-management courses.

The medical care of individuals with RA mirrors the general shift in Western industrial societies from acute care to the management and treatment of chronic illness. This has posed a considerable challenge to health care professionals and led to an increasing focus on the psychological and social aspects surrounding chronic illnesses as the day-to-day management increasingly falls on the individual and her family. This is particularly the case in a disease like RA which involves major psychological adaptation. Individuals with RA face the prospect of a lifetime of a painful and increasingly disabling illness without the prospect of a cure, having to take regular medication and face the possibility of major surgery for joint replacement sometime in their lives. The adaptive tasks required of someone with RA not only involve coming to terms with the symptoms and treatment but also adapting to altered life plans, reduced employment prospects and perhaps the most difficult challenge of dealing with the uncertainty regarding the course of the disease. It is the lifetime and ever-changing adaptation required that makes RA a disease that can place great stress on the individual as well as on friends and families. In the early stages of the disease before a diagnosis has been confirmed individuals have to attempt to understand what the symptoms mean to them. Later, it will not always be straightforward or easy to predict what the future course of their illness will be. What is important is that despite the stress that most individuals with RA have to face, the majority rise to these challenges and deal with the problems of the illness and its lack of cure.

In order to understand how individuals think and behave in response to their RA it is necessary to consider how they interpret and understand their own symptoms, what theories they develop regarding the causes and treatments of RA, what they may be able to do about their symptoms and the course of the disease. These cognitions will not only guide their behaviour but are likely to be communicated to others in their environment. Their cognitions and those of those around them are also likely to reflect the general attitudes and beliefs in the society regarding sickness and health.

The dominant symptoms of RA are pain and stiffness. Like all symptoms they need to be understood from both a biological and a psychological perspective. For the individual with RA the impact of pain is to restrict activities. This frequently sets up a cascade of effects all of which serve to increase the stress placed on the individual with RA. The most direct impact is on the type and amount of work individuals can undertake. In many cases constraints regarding work derive from an inflexibility in organisation and structure in the work environment which tends to be unimaginative in responding to disability. The work restrictions in turn have a significant effect on income which in turn restricts activities and the ability to recruit assistance. It also serves to reduce social interaction and thus increases the likelihood of social isolation. Individuals who are isolated have a reduced opportunity to call on others for both practical and emotional help or support. The establishment of self-help and support groups has gone some way to counter this trend.

One of the features of RA is that it affects women disproportionately to men in a ratio of approximately 3 to 1. It is common nowadays for women to combine paid employment with child-rearing and on both of these RA appears to impose restrictions for many women. Because of the increased incidence of RA in women it frequently falls on the men to perform the role of carer. While all carers find themselves in roles that they did not expect to perform, this may be especially so for many men. This alteration of roles and the stresses that arise from being a carer emphasise the pervasive influence of RA.

One of the main sources of information and advice regarding RA comes from physicians. The communication between doctors and patients is important for both patient satisfaction and adherence to medical advice and medication. In RA the patients are often experienced in the illness and its effects and consequently a successful model of care needs to take account of the patient's perceptions and cognitions about the illness and treatment.

Most of the time people with RA have to cope with their illness themselves. It is important to understand how some individuals appear to succeed in dealing very well with the disease whilst others have great difficulty. The findings of studies of how people cope with their RA have been used as the basis for planning educational, psychological and social interventions. Their efficacy has led to these approaches being seen as an important adjunct to medical interventions.

The real challenge for a comprehensive understanding of RA is not only to take account of medical knowledge but to comprehensively embrace a model which incorporates the psychological and social factors related to the illness. It is through this biopsychosocial approach that we will be best able to understand RA. This book is an attempt to present developments in some psychological and social domains in order to contribute to the development of a broad-based understanding of RA.

ORGANISATION OF THIS VOLUME

In Chapter 2 we present the nature of RA and its treatment to provide the medical and epidemiological background to the following chapters. This chapter also indicates some of the rationale for writing a whole book on the psychological and social factors around one illness. The high incidence of RA, its lifelong nature, its variable and unpredictable course for most individuals and its disabling consequences all combine to make an understanding of the individual's experience of RA important for health care professionals.

Chapter 3 presents the experience of RA from the patient's perspective. This important approach to the understanding of illness is one which has traditionally not had much attention until recent years. Considering patients' views enables an appreciation of the meaning of the illness and its treatment to individuals from their own point of view. What issues concern individuals with RA at different stages of the illness, how they understand the causes of RA, and how they deal with their social roles are all examined in this chapter. This chapter and Chapter 2 are intended to provide the background from both a medical and personal perspective for the following chapters.

The dominant symptoms of RA, pain and stiffness, are discussed in Chapter 4. These are covered from both the biological and psychological perspectives.

In Chapter 5 we examine the impact RA has on quality of life and how the various aspects of quality of life are measured. This chapter is intended to provide an understanding of the different measures used in arthritis and also to examine the evidence regarding the impact of RA on psychological and social functioning.

The central question of Chapter 6 asks what the patient might expect from encounters with the doctor. Much information about illness is obtained through the doctor and we present how different factors in this important interaction for any individual with RA may influence subsequent behaviour and experience. As most individuals with RA are women and more men than women are physicians the issue of gender and its influence on the interaction between patient and doctor is picked up as an important theme in this chapter.

Chapter 7 considers how far our understanding of what patients do in the face of their RA influences the course of the illness and their well-being. How patients cope with their illness has been an issue of concern for social scientists for some time and this chapter examines the ways in which the term 'coping' has been conceptualised and assessed within RA and the extent to which there is an understanding that certain forms of coping lead to better outcomes.

The context of coping with a chronic illness such as RA is examined in Chapter 8. Within RA much research has been performed on the construct of social support. This chapter examines the importance of social support for individuals with RA and presents a number of different theoretical frameworks. The importance of the spouse of the individual with RA and the role of support groups are presented here in order to gain an appreciation of the widespread influence of RA beyond the patient.

The final chapter focuses on psychological interventions in RA. The treatment of pain in RA can be tackled with both traditional pharmacological intervention as well as psychological approaches. In the final chapter the major psychological and educational interventions and their efficacy in RA are presented.

Certain topics permeate the book. These include in particular depression and psychological well-being in arthritis. As many of the measured outcomes as well as some interventions relate to psychological well-being, this issue is covered in most of the chapters.

The book does not attempt to be comprehensive and there are specific areas which have not been addressed. These include, for example, work on the important relationship between the stresses of RA and the immune system. In addition no attempt has been made to present models of stress and psychological functioning. These topics may well be the focus of a future volume on RA.

While the book attempts to provide a current overview of the psychological and social factors in RA it is important to bear in mind that this is a growing field for social science researchers and our knowledge and understanding is set to increase in future years. As medical treatments change and new approaches become available so the issues that individuals face will change and our current understanding of the experience of RA will need to be revised.

Chapter 2

The disorder and its treatment

Despite a great deal of basic clinical research, little is known about the causes of rheumatoid arthritis (RA) and no cures have yet been discovered. It will become clear from this chapter that drugs and other therapies are intended largely to reduce the symptoms of RA and arrest the progress of underlying disease. To develop goals and targets for the health care of individuals with RA it is necessary to have a long-term view of the disease over the whole life-course. Also there is a distinct social distribution to RA; women are more likely to have RA than men and individuals with fewer educational and socioeconomic resources experience more problems arising from RA. This social patterning is a major challenge to our understanding of the illness and ultimately to how we provide care.

THE NATURE OF RHEUMATOID ARTHRITIS

Rheumatoid arthritis is a chronic inflammatory disease that affects the synovial tissue surrounding the joints. This inflammation is associated with swelling and pain. As the disease progresses joint tissue may become permanently damaged. The combined effects of inflammation and joint damage result in progressive disability. RA is one of a range of rheumatic and musculo-skeletal disorders that includes osteoarthritis, ankylosing spondylitis, various conditions resulting in back pain, arthritis, fibromyalgia and lupus erythrematosus, and increasingly precise definitions and clinical criteria have been sought to distinguish RA from these related disorders (Rigby and Wood, 1990). Currently the diagnostic criteria of the American College of Rheumatology are widely recommended, although clinicians are not confined to these criteria in making diagnoses (Table 2.1). The criteria for diagnosis involve clinical signs of disease activity in the joints, together with evidence from x-rays and the presence of rheumatoid factor from serum. Rheumatoid factor is a form of antibody to type II collagen. It is suggested that these antibodies are evidence of auto-immune responses that bring about the disease. Although this evidence is by no means clear, the presence of rheumatoid factor has for a long time been considered an important diagnostic variable. However, in some recent studies it has become clear that as many as 72 per cent of those who have a positive test for rheumatoid factor may not have the disease (Shmerling and Delbanco, 1992).

Table 2.1 Criteria for the classification of rheumatoid arthritis

Four or more of the following should be present:

- Morning stiffness
- Arthritis of three or more joint areas
- Arthritis of hand joints
- Symmetrical arthritis
- Rheumatoid nodules
- Serum rheumatoid factor
- Radiographic changes

Source: Arnett *et al.* (1987)

Osteoarthritis is far more common than rheumatoid arthritis. The presence of osteoarthritis can be detected in over 80 per cent of individuals beyond the age of 75 years. It used to be commonly referred to as 'wear and tear' arthritis because it is often induced by injury or excess use of joints. It is a disease that affects joint cartilage and the underlying bone. It initially affects smaller joints but eventually involves major weight-bearing joints such as the hip or knee.

The causes of RA are, as yet, unknown. It is generally considered an auto-immune disease, but there is no clear evidence of what factors trigger this destructive response of the body's immune system. Some research evidence supports the view that a virus such as Epstein-Barr may be involved in the initial triggering of the auto-immune response that leads to RA. However, it is also possible that such phenomena are secondary to the onset of RA (Sewell and Trentham, 1993). It does appear that, however triggered, T-cells, which are normally part of the body's adaptive immune system and which normally respond against foreign bodies, are induced to attack the individual's joints (Harris, 1990). There is also evidence that these auto-immune responses more commonly occur in individuals who are genetically susceptible. Twin studies to assess concordance for risks of RA have, to date, been inconclusive, but do provide some evidence of a heritable component (Aho *et al.*, 1986).

The course of RA

At the very beginning, when antigens are presented to susceptible individuals, the disease is usually silent and without symptoms. For the majority of individuals, the onset of symptoms is gradual and insidious. However, for a minority of approximately 10–15 per cent onset may be quite rapid with quite severe symptoms developing over a few days or weeks. For all, early symptoms are a product of the inflammation of joints. Initially, symptoms are more likely to affect the hands and wrists. In these stages individuals experience the pain, swelling and stiffness that are the cardinal characteristics of the disease, but may also feel fatigue and general malaise (Liang *et al.*, 1992).

The long-term course of RA is so highly varied among individuals as to defy description of any single pattern. However, it is possible to distinguish three different trajectories (Scott and Huskisson, 1992). By far the most common pattern, found in approximately 70 per cent of diagnosed individuals, is progressive disease with periodic fluctuations of flares and remissions. A second, much less common pattern (25 per cent) is intermittent, with episodes of RA flares and brief intermissions. A small proportion of this second pattern experience much longer periods of intermission. A third quite uncommon group (less than 5 per cent) experience what is termed 'malignant' disease, an extremely severe form. For the majority of individuals the course of RA involves periodic 'flare-ups', episodes when the disease is more active and symptoms more severe.

When RA does progress, the disease invades the cartilage, tendons and bone and the irreversible destruction of tissue begins to occur. An increasing number of joints begin to be affected. Joint erosion may actually begin within the first two years of onset of the disease (Brook and Corbett, 1971). At later stages of the disease, progressive destruction of joints occurs. As joint damage becomes greater, the patient becomes increasingly disabled.

The long-term outcome of RA also varies. Overall there is a common pattern of increased disability. Sherrer and colleagues (1986) studied the course of RA in 681 patients recruited from a wide range of clinics in Saskatchewan. They observed that patients' disability developed more rapidly during the first few years after onset and that disability increased subsequently but at a relatively slower rate. Using a standardised rating of functional class (Steinbrocker *et al.*, 1949), 88 per cent of patients were in the two less disabled groups (Class I 'complete functional capacity' and Class II 'functional capacity adequate to conduct normal activities despite handicap of discomfort or limited mobility of one or more joints'). Only 9 per cent of patients were in Class III ('functional capacity quite limited'), and 3 per cent in Class IV ('largely or wholly incapacitated'). Eleven years later, the proportions of the sample in these two most severe classes had increased to 19 per cent and 16 per cent respectively. A British hospital study also illustrates the progressive disability found in RA but suggests a somewhat different medium-term course (Scott *et al.*, 1987). This sample of 112 patients appeared to be a much more disabled group at the beginning of the study than the Saskatchewan study, with 77 per cent of the sample placed in the two most impaired groups according to Steinbrocker criteria. After 10 years this figure had dropped to 46 per cent; indicating that the sample had become somewhat less disabled. However after 20 years of follow-up, the proportion of severely disabled amongst survivors had risen again to 82 per cent.

Other studies confirm an overall trend of progressively increased disability, but vary in the picture presented of the rate at which such deterioration occurs, the extent of disability at outcome and whether there is accelerated deterioration early in the history of the disease (Wolfe and Cathey, 1991; Rasker and Cosh 1992; Leigh and Fries, 1992). The lack of agreement across studies may be accounted for largely by variations in sample recruitment, length of time for which patients are followed, measurement error and degree of success in maintaining cohorts in the study. In several of the studies, the initial level of disability was a strong predictor of degree of disability at the end of the study (Wolfe and Cathey, 1991; Leigh and Fries, 1992). The influence of patients' initial disease and disability on patterns of outcome is not surprising.

It may also be possible that existing measures of disability provide misleading evidence of the extent of progression in disability associated with RA. Gardiner and colleagues (1993) followed up 245 patients with RA over a period of 5 years. As in other studies, they found that patients experienced serious deterioration in disability over this time period. They also noted, however, that patients who at the beginning of the study had the most severe disability as measured by the Health Assessment Questionnaire (HAQ; Fries *et al.*, 1982), deteriorated very little in the subsequent 5 years despite the fact that the majority reported that their RA was worse at follow-up than at baseline. By contrast, patients with more favourable HAQ scores at baseline also tended to say that their RA had deteriorated 5 years later, but showed a marked deterioration. The authors suggest that such findings may arise through 'ceiling effects' in the measurement of disability via the HAQ. The instrument does not leave room for the most disabled individuals to report further deterioration. Thus, given that most cohort studies have used the HAQ or other similar instruments to assess outcomes in terms of disability, overall deterioration may have been minimised. The measurement of disability is discussed in a subsequent chapter (see Chapter 5).

It used to be commonly observed that RA, whilst a very disabling disease, was never fatal. It is no longer possible to be so reassuring. Only one of ten studies reviewed by Pinals (1987) failed to observe excess mortality in patients with RA compared with the general population. In one sample of patients with RA, deaths were considered by clinicians to be directly related to the disease in 19 per cent of the cases, indirectly related in another 14 per cent and unrelated in the majority (66 per cent). The relationship of mortality to the disease was largely attributed to systemic effects of the disease, rather than side-effects of drugs (Rasker and Cosh, 1992). A similar study examining deaths in patients with RA over a 20 year period also interpreted deaths as more likely to be caused by systemic effects of disease than side-effects of drugs (Scott *et al.*, 1987). It is increasingly argued that the long-term 'side-effects' of the disease must be balanced against possible side-effects of drugs in planning treatment (Pincus and Callahan, 1993a).

CURRENT TREATMENTS

Treatment of RA is concerned with arresting the development of the disease and associated disability and reducing the severity of symptoms. As the causes of RA have not been identified, therapies are somewhat indirect in their mode of action, aimed at reducing joint inflammation and swelling and consequently pain, stiffness and joint deterioration. The most common forms of therapy are pharmacological, although increasingly attention is being given to alternative forms of treatment including physical therapy, wearing splints or paraffin baths that will reduce the consequences of the disease. Many of the pharmacological treatments can have quite toxic effects so the choice and monitoring of drug treatments in relation to costs and benefits is complex.

Drug treatments for RA are considered either 'symptomatic' or 'slow-acting antirheumatic' (the latter are often also referred to as 'disease-modifying' or 'second line'). Symptomatic drugs are not intended to have any impact on underlying disease processes. Symptomatic treatment requires the use of one or more of the wide class of non-steroidal anti-inflammatory drugs (NSAIDs) (such as aspirin or ibuprofen) which are intended to reduce the severity of inflammation and stiffness experienced by the patient. Analgesics may also be used to control pain. One major problem with NSAIDs is that they are one of the commonest sources of adverse reactions (Brooks, 1993). The most common reaction is in gastrointestinal upset but other problems such as renal or skin damage may occur. There seems to be no clear evidence to support the use of any particular NSAID in preference to others (Joint Working Group, 1992).

If the disease is very active or shows no response to NSAIDs, treatment in the form of slow-acting antirheumatic drugs (SAARDs) will be tried. These drugs are chemically very diverse and have a wide range of modes of action that may result in arresting disease progression but have no direct analgesic properties (Dawes and Symmons, 1992). As with NSAIDs, the choice of drug is complex and all SAARDs have potential side-effects. A recent meta-analysis of clinical trials identified gold injections, D-penicillamine, sulphasalazine and methotrexate as having more favourable evidence for effectiveness than orally ingested gold or chloroquine (Felson *et al.*, 1990). Some have advocated that, to be fully effective, SAARDs need to be introduced at a much earlier phase in the history of RA than has hitherto been the usual practice (Wilske and Healey, 1989). Currently there is no agreement about the merits of this approach especially as it can expose patients needlessly to serious side-effects of drugs. There is a yet more powerful class of so-called 'third-line drugs' such as azathioprine to be used when SAARDs have failed. However this class is cytotoxic, and risks in relation to benefits are not at all clear; third-line drugs tend to be recommended for patients with the most severe and active forms of the disease and the poorest prognosis (Porter and Sturrock, 1993).

Several studies have suggested that long-term outcomes of pharmacological management of RA are not very favourable. One problem which considerably reduces the potential longer-term benefits of drugs is that many patients withdraw or are removed from their prescribed course of treatment because of side-effects. In one study, by 6 months 23 per cent of patients had given up their drug regime of injected gold, 27 per cent had given up azathioprine, and 48 per cent cyclophosphamide (Singh *et al.*, 1991). In another study Wolfe and colleagues (1990) estimated that the average length of time that patients could remain on SAARDs was one and a half to two years. Apart from diminishing therapeutic benefits, the short 'life-span' of most drug regimens adds a further difficulty to the many other logistic problems of conducting long-term trials. Consequently, although a number of trials demonstrate the benefits of SAARDs over one or two years, there is little evidence to support the view that they have long-term effects in slowing the rate of disease progression or arresting disability (Rasker and Cosh, 1992). Indeed the more disappointing long-term outcomes for RA reported earlier in this chapter appear to reflect the current efficacy of pharmacological treatment.

Individuals with RA may also benefit from surgery. This may involve carpel tunnel surgery to relieve compression of nerves in the wrist caused by arthritis. Far more common is the replacement of major joints, particularly the hip and knee. This step may be considered with individuals experiencing particularly severe pain and disability. Most joint-replacement surgery is performed for individuals with osteoarthritis. Decisions regarding appropriateness of joint-replacement surgery for younger individuals with rheumatoid arthritis can be difficult because replacement joints may last only 15 years before requiring further replacement and such revisions are very difficult.

Complementary medicine

In their search for relief from pain and disability individuals with arthritis often resort to complementary remedies. Problems with joints, including backs, are the main complaint amongst people seeking help from complementary sources (Sharma 1992). A study of patients attending a rheumatology clinic in Birmingham, Alabama found that 94 per cent of respondents had used at least one form of unorthodox therapy for their arthritis (Kronenfeld and Wasner, 1982). Over 80 per cent of respondents had used topical remedies such as liniments or ointments. Fifty four per cent had used some form of special diet and 38 per cent tried wearing copper or some other form of jewellery. In another study (Cronan *et al.*, 1989), 84 per cent had used one or more unconventional therapies.

A voluntary association for individuals with rheumatic diseases in the UK, Arthritis Care, carried out a survey of its members (Arthritis Care, 1989). The most commonly used non-orthodox medicines were fish-oil-based preparations (28 per cent) and a range of vitamins and herbal remedies (16 per cent). They also reported use of complementary practitioners. Sixteen per cent had consulted an osteopath and 12 per cent an acupuncturist. The use of complementary therapy and the extent of benefits derived have not been examined.

Issues in assessing treatment efficacy

It is important to stress that two patients may end up at the same level of disability 25 or 30 years after the onset of illness whilst their illness trajectories may have varied enormously, with one patient having experienced much less pain and disability and a more favourable quality of life in the intervening period. Thus, although long-term-outcome studies are currently disappointing, the scope for improving immediate and intermediate outcomes is enormous. For this reason the scope for improvement to be obtained from the range of cognitive, educational and social-support-based therapies discussed later in the volume becomes as vital to assess as the pharmacological interventions discussed here.

One problem that is faced in any attempt to assess the effectiveness of therapies is that a wide range of measures of outcome are used in clinical trials of RA. There has been no consensus as to which are the most important or more informative of the many radiological, laboratory, clinical and patient-based measures. The result has been that studies differ quite markedly in how they assess outcomes, making comparisons across studies difficult. A recent consensus conference (Felson *et al.*, 1993) has identified a core set of measures recommended for use in all clinical trials (Table 2.2). It is quite noticeable how important are the patient's own judgements of the disease and its impact on function.

Table 2.2 American College of Rheumatology core set of measures of disease activity for clinical trials in rheumatoid arthritis

- Tender joint count
- Swollen joint count
- Patient's assessment of pain
- Patient's global assessment of disease activity
- Doctor's global assessment of disease activity
- Patient's assessment of physical function (e.g. with HAQ)
- Acute phase reactant value (e.g. ESR)

(for longer term trials)

- Radiographic evidence

Source: Felson *et al.* (1993)

THE EPIDEMIOLOGY OF RA

Arthritis and rheumatism as a whole are the biggest single source of disability in UK and North American populations. If one takes self-reports of arthritis, 29 per cent of men and 32 per cent of women in a US national survey reported symptoms possibly related to arthritis such as pain, swelling and morning stiffness in joints (Cunningham and Kelsey, 1984). Other surveys have produced similarly high rates (Holbrook *et al.*, 1990). A nationwide survey in the USA of adults aged 55 or older, produced an even higher prevalence of self-reported arthritis: 35 per cent of men and 51 per cent of women (Verbrugge *et al.*, 1991). These estimates depend on individuals' own definitions of their symptoms and group together all forms of arthritis and musculoskeletal disease. Estimates of the prevalence of RA are much lower but vary considerably according to the definition of the disorder used. Figures for the prevalence of RA range from 1 per cent to 3 per cent of the population with lower estimates obtained when studies rely on x-ray data and medical examination (Verbrugge *et al.*, 1991). Overall, both European and North American surveys that use more rigorous definitions of RA show a remarkable degree of convergence in estimates of prevalence varying between 0.8 per cent and 1.0 per cent (Wood and Badley, 1986).

There is evidence of some geographical variation in the prevalence of RA. Thus, some Chinese and African populations have a lower prevalence of the disorder than is found in European or American populations (Wood and Badley, 1986; Lau *et al.*, 1993). Additionally a lower prevalence of RA among Black Caribbeans compared with whites has recently been reported in one British city (MacGregor *et al.*, 1994). However these variations are not well understood and have not provided any helpful insights into the causation of RA. Overall the evidence from epidemiology is more striking for the uniformity of rates between geographical regions.

The rate of new cases of RA in the population, the incidence rate, has been shown to increase with age in all studies. In a survey of RA among women in Seattle, Washington, at ages 30–39, the incidence per 100,000 was 16.5, and by ages 60–64, the rate had nearly quadrupled – 61.6 per 100,000 (Dugowson *et al.*, 1991). The association of RA with older age is two-fold; the risk of onset increases with ageing and the disability associated with the disease increases over time (Scott and Huskisson, 1992).

There is some encouraging evidence from both the US and the UK that the incidence of RA has begun to decline among women but not among men (Spector 1991). Also observed are some changes in the nature of disease. Anderson and colleagues (1990) have noted that over time the proportion of patients in more severe classes of the disease has declined. At present data are not sufficiently conclusive and reasons for any decline in incidence and severity are quite speculative. It has, for example, been suggested that such changes in the character of the disease are consistent with a viral aetiology (Spector, 1991).

The influence of gender

One of the most striking features of RA is that it is far more common in women. The reasons for this pattern are not well understood and represent an important challenge to research. To begin with, the exact nature of the difference in prevalence is unclear. Overall, the most commonly agreed estimate is of a female/male ratio of 3:1. However, if one only examines patients within a year of onset of the disease, the differences in rates between men and women disappear (Fleming *et al.*, 1976). This has led to the suggestion that RA has a similar incidence in men and women, but that there is more remission among men and the course of the disease is less severe (Da Silva and Hall, 1992). It has also been observed that there are much smaller differences in rates of the onset of the disease beyond the ages of 60 (Inoue *et al.*, 1987). Thus it has been suggested that the overall pattern of a much higher prevalence in women is due to an earlier age of onset in women, typically 45–64, and a more severe course (Da Silva and Hall, 1992).

Much of the evidence supports the view that women experience RA in a more severe form than men, but it is not all consistent. In terms of conventional rheumatological measures, Carvalho and colleagues (1980) found from radiological evidence that women had more severe damage in the hands from RA than did men, but there were no differences for large joints. In another study women appeared more severely affected by RA according to clinical assessment of joint damage but there were no differences in terms of laboratory (ESR) or radiographic evidence (Caruso *et al.*, 1990). Pathria and colleagues (1988) could find no differences by gender for severity of disease as measured by x-ray in a sample of men and women matched for age and disease duration.

In addition to assessing gender differences in RA by means of rheumatological measures, differences in the personal impact of the disease also need to be considered. A number of studies have examined gender differences by means of the Health Assessment Questionnaire (Fries *et al.*, 1982) which provides an assessment of disability arising from RA. The majority of these studies indicate greater disability for women (Ekdahl *et al.*, 1988; Thompson and Pegley, 1991; Deighton *et al.*, 1992). Studies using other instruments to assess the impact of RA also indicate greater impact for women, in areas such as energy and fatigue (Fitzpatrick, Ziebland, *et al.*, 1992), mobility (Spiegel *et al.*, 1988) and pain (Weinberger *et al.*, 1986). In some comparative studies the greatest differences are found in areas of domestic work such as cleaning and shopping (Verbrugge *et al.*, 1991; Reisine and Fifield, 1992). However not all studies support this pattern of gender differences (Guillemin *et al.*, 1992).

For the most part, these studies concentrate on cross-sectional gender differences in the severity of RA. Another perspective is obtained by examining changes over time in the course of RA. Several such longitudinal studies suggest that women may have a poorer long-term outcome (Da Silva and Hall, 1992). Leigh and Fries (1992) followed 330 individuals with RA over an 8 year period. After controlling for a variety of measures of disease severity and age at baseline, gender was one of the most important predictors of subsequent disability as measured by self-report on the HAQ. In a similarly designed study of 681 patients with RA followed up over nearly 12 years, gender was again the most important predictor of outcome in terms of disability on the HAQ, after measures of disease severity and age (Sherrer *et al.*, 1986). In both studies women experienced less favourable outcomes. However other studies have not found significant differences between men and women in the course of RA. Thus in Gardiner *et al.*'s (1993) study of 245 patients followed up over 5 years, women had initially poorer HAQ scores but gender failed to predict long-term outcome. Poorer prognoses for women in terms of disability have to be compared with the greater mortality experienced by men. In two major longitudinal studies over 5 years (Kazis *et al.*, 1990) and 8 years (Leigh and Fries, 1991), men were found to have significantly higher mortality rates, independently of other predictors.

Reasons for these observed differences in prevalence between men and women are not understood despite considerable research efforts to examine a wide range of underlying mechanisms. The most obvious biological explanations have focused on reproductive hormones such as testosterone and oestrogen. Such influences would account for the common observation that women experience temporary remission from RA symptoms during pregnancy (Klipple and Cecere, 1989). Moreover it has been suggested that there is a possible beneficial effect of oral contraceptives (Vandenbroucke *et al.*, 1982). It has been suggested that oral contraceptives reduce the incidence of RA by postponing its onset which often occurs once the oral contraceptive has been stopped (Spector and Hochberg, 1990).

There is a variety of ways in which reproductive hormones might influence the causes or course of RA. There are, for example, many complex relationships between hormones and the immune system. Reproductive hormones may also have a direct influence on cartilage. However research evidence regarding the relationship between reproductive hormones and RA is contradictory and inconclusive. For example, where evidence is found of elevated levels of a hormone in patients with RA, it may well be that the elevation is a consequence rather than a cause of the disease (Da Silva and Hall, 1992). Even more speculative at this stage are suggestions of gender differences in the HLA antigen system. The HLA antigen system is generally considered to be implicated in the aetiology of RA, but there is no clear evidence of gender differences in its expression.

A number of alternative explanations have been offered to account for gender differences in disability resulting from RA. The simplest explanation is that women experience more disability because of the more severe and aggressive form of the disease that they experience. A number of studies have attempted to examine this possibility by determining whether differences in disability between men and women persist if level of disease severity is controlled for. Unfortunately results have been contradictory, with one study finding that at comparable levels of disease activity women's disability is worse (Thompson and Pegley, 1991), whereas in another study, differences in disability disappear after controlling for disease severity (Deighton *et al.*, 1992). A related possibility is that other aspects of health and fitness that differ between men and women may result in greater disability for women after the onset of RA. For example, Verbrugge and colleagues (1991) found that one of the biggest differences between men and women with arthritis was (self-reported) strength; thus, performing the same tasks or daily activities may pose a greater challenge for women than for men.

Problems of interpreting differences in self-reported illness and disability between men and women are not confined to RA. In both the UK and USA, surveys find higher levels of morbidity (symptoms), days of restriction due to illness and visits to the doctor among women (Waldron, 1983). The interpretation of such differences has proved controversial. Many explanations treat the differences as 'real' and seek mechanisms to explain them. Interpretations have focused on biological processes that may vary between men and women and specific risk-taking behaviours that lead to impaired health. Alternatively, particularly in the field of psychiatric illness, explanations for 'real' gender differences in psychological well-being are sought either in differential socialisation patterns for men and women, different sets of social stresses and different social roles and statuses (Gove and Tudor, 1973). Some studies have pointed to the multiple roles women occupy in modern Western societies and the strain this places upon their health (Arber, 1990).

An opposing viewpoint encompasses explanations for gender differences in self-reported morbidity which argue that the differences are not 'real'. Women's roles are said to leave more time to consult for health problems (Miles, 1991), and women find it easier to reveal problems and seek help than men (Briscoe, 1982). Women are more health aware and have higher expectations in relation to health (Mechanic, 1976). It has also been argued that instruments for eliciting symptoms, health problems or level of disability may have a built-in gender bias so that more female forms of problem are identified, a form of argument that is actually quite difficult to prove or disprove (Tousignant *et al.*, 1987).

Other research has focused less on the over-recognition of womens' health problems and more on problems of under-recognition. Reisine and colleagues (1987) have argued that many aspects of the impact of RA in women are less well recognised because of the ways in which disability is conventionally assessed in contemporary society. In particular, whilst the impact of RA on instrumental activities such as shopping and cooking are increasingly incorporated into assessments, other forms of domestic activity, 'nurturant functions' such as childcare, caring for sick members of the household and maintaining the social contacts of the household with wider social networks are not included. As many women are not employed in paid occupations, and even if they are, view domestic roles as a central part of their lives, current approaches to disability systematically downplay the impact of RA in this respect (Williams, 1987). In a sample of 142 women with classical or definite RA (Reisine *et al.*, 1987), 72 per cent of the women reported some limitation in at least one nurturant function, most commonly problems arising from RA in their ability to maintain the family's social ties and social arrangements (42 per cent), in looking after family members when sick (39 per cent) or in childcare (29 per cent).

In a subsequent study, Reisine and Fifield (1992) examined further the possible problems for women with RA arising from currently limited definitions of disability. In a study of 998 patients with RA recruited from 56 randomly selected clinics throughout the USA, they found that women experienced higher levels of disability arising from RA compared with men and were more likely to report being unable to undertake paid work because of RA. However women were also *less* likely to receive social security benefits because of loss of paid work. The most likely reasons for such discrepancies is that entitlement to benefits is limited by patterns of work history prior to onset of disability and women's employment histories may have made them less eligible. In the same study Reisine and Fifield also found that whereas women reported more physical limitations arising from RA than men, they were *less* likely than the men in the sample to be assessed as severely disabled by their doctors. In terms of access to social benefits and medical recognition of disability, women may be disadvantaged. Both problems indicate the considerable scope for social and cultural definitions of disability to influence the course of RA.

Above all, this broader literature on gender differences in health has revealed and increasingly emphasised the heterogeneity of women's experience concealed by gender categories. Differences of social background, employment status and social support among other factors may have substantial influences on health status. Indeed, one body of evidence demonstrates that when the social circumstances of women and men are most similar, gender differences in psychiatric rates disappear (Jenkins and Clare, 1985). It is possible that a similar phenomenon has yet to be uncovered with rheumatoid arthritis.

Socioeconomic status

In looking at general patterns of morbidity and mortality in Britain and other Western societies, the influence of social class on health is unequivocal. The effects of class have been clearly demonstrated in relation to a range of social variables including occupation, income, education and housing (Townsend *et al.*, 1988; Davey Smith and Egger 1993). However, in general, evidence for an association between social class and both the occurrence and outcome of musculoskeletal disorders is patchy.

There have been occasional reports that the risk of developing RA is inversely related to income and occupational status (King and Cobb 1958; Engel 1968). However, very few studies have examined the issue systematically since the studies of miners in the 1950s (Miall *et al.*, 1953). The majority of reports suggest that there is no overall relationship with social class (Lawrence 1970; Jacob *et al.*, 1972). More recently, however, it has been suggested that patient behaviours and lifestyle, identified through the marker of 'formal educational level' appear to be significant and under-recognised influences on the prevalence of RA (Pincus and Callahan 1993b). With regard to specific occupational factors, there is little other than anecdotal evidence for the association between particular activities within occupations and aches and pains in different joints. There is anecdotal evidence also to suggest that joints stressed at work may become more severely damaged by RA (Wood and Badley 1986), but no evidence of any overall connection between RA and occupation.

Of more interest to social scientists may be the existence of any evidence for an association between socioeconomic status and health outcomes in RA. Again, the evidence is hard to come by. The natural history of RA continues to confound those working in the field (Pincus and Callahan 1993a). However, evidence from the USA does suggest that 'formal education' is an important predictor of both morbidity and mortality in RA (Pincus and Callahan 1985, 1986). Among a sample of 75 patients, the 9-year survival rate was 95 per cent in patients with more than 12 years' formal education, 71 per cent in patients with 9–12 years, and 55 per cent in those with 8 or fewer years of formal education. The mean levels of decline in functional status were 22 per cent, 29 per cent, and 58 per cent respectively in these groups. Of the patients with fewer than 8 years' education 75 per cent experienced the poorest two outcomes of death or a 50 per cent loss of functional status, compared with only 25 per cent of the patients with 12 or more years of education (Pincus and Callahan 1986). Clearly, the questions of what 'education' is an indicator of in these circumstances, and what may mediate its effects on RA, remain moot and deserve further study. However, these studies stand as an important attempt to link rheumatic disease epidemiology to broader concerns within social epidemiology.

In the UK, a study of mortality in RA (Prior *et al.*, 1984) did give rise to correspondence which raised the issue of the role of social class in mortality in RA (Lyle 1984; Prior and Symmons 1984). However, the jury remains out and the authors of the study conclude:

> Whatever the true distribution of social class in individuals with RA, we conclude that the distribution in our series did not invalidate the use of national statistics in our analysis and that the demonstrated excess of some causes of death was not due entirely to social class.
>
> (Prior and Symmons 1984: 10)

If one adopts a broader definition of outcome than is typically employed in clinical epidemiological studies, RA does appear to be more disabling for working-class than for middle-class people, although interpretation of these findings is difficult (Liang *et al.*, 1981). Twenty-five years ago it was shown that sickness absence due to 'rheumatism' was twice as high in dockers as in civil servants (Partridge and Duthie 1968). Other studies indicated that the speed with which someone with RA returned to work after treatment was affected by both education and work background (Robins and Walters 1971). More recently the work of Yelin and his colleagues, in a series of both cross-sectional and longitudinal studies, has indicated that social and workplace factors are more predictive of work disability among individuals with RA than are disease factors (Yelin *et al.*, 1980; 1986; 1987). These workplace influences on disability include not only the physical requirements of jobs but also the worker's discretion regarding the pace and scheduling of work tasks.

Systematic attempts to explore the relationship between social class and RA are scarce. In general, epidemiologists seem to have little interest in the matter; another illustration, perhaps, of the curious research priorities within rheumatology (Williams *et al.*, 1992).

SUMMARY

Rheumatoid arthritis is a chronic inflammatory disease of unknown causes. The impact of the disease on individuals varies as does its course over time. None of the wide variety of treatments available is capable of reversing or curing the disease. There are puzzling differences in the pattern of RA by gender and social background.

Chapter 3

The experience of rheumatoid arthritis

INTRODUCTION

Medicine is primarily concerned with disease. A glance at any of the classical texts – in the Western world at least – reveals the same basic pattern in terms of which the formal knowledge of the specialty is organised. In the same fashion, the specialist journals publish articles dealing with nosology, aetiology, treatment, mortality and so forth as they relate to particular diseases. In all of this work the disease, be it back pain, rheumatoid arthritis, or systemic lupus erythematosus, is defined as an objective entity which, with study and research, can be understood better and treated more effectively.

This perspective is sometimes referred to as 'the biomedical model'. What has been lacking from this traditional model of disease is a means of understanding the experiences of those who have the disease (Engel, 1977). In this, rheumatology is no exception to the general rule. While rheumatology textbooks have increasingly included within their contents chapters or sections on the psychological or social aspects of a disease (Scott, 1986; Kelley *et al.*, 1993; Maddison *et al.*, 1993), these have been written for the most part by doctors or other health professionals as they see the impact upon their patients. Patients have been excluded both because their own subjective viewpoint was thought to be marginal to the treatment process, and because being subjective was thought to compromise that objectivity which is the *sine qua non* of medical knowledge. The more sophisticated biological explanations for disease have become, the more difficult it has been to relate these to the experience of the individual concerned (Comaroff and Maguire, 1981).

Prior to the early 1980s, work on the experience of illness, of what it was like to be sick in society, was quite rare (Schneider and Conrad, 1983). In more recent times, however, this situation has changed. The traditional focus on the disease separately from the experience and situation of the person who has the disease has come to be questioned for three reasons.

First, sociologists, anthropologists and psychologists have, in different ways, tried to look at the disorder from the patient's point of view. Rather than focusing on the disease, such work has underlined the importance of the way in which diseases are experienced as illnesses and are situated as handicaps. It seeks to understand the meaning of illness *for* the individual by grasping the *consequences* of the disease. This work also seeks to understand the meaning of the illness *to* the individual in as much as it seeks to understand the *significance* of bodily changes (Bury, 1991). Methodologically these represent two levels of analysis in the study of chronic disease: one focusing on the personal and social problems which intrude on everyday life; the other highlighting the manner in which those problems are integrated within an account or narrative (Williams, 1993). The goal of these analyses taken together is to understand the way individual people live with illnesses in social contexts, and to consider its implication for the treatments and services they receive.

Second, one of the most profound developments in Western societies over the last 50 years or so has been the shift in the age structure of the population. This means that there is likely to be a steady and disproportionate increase in the numbers of people requiring treatment for various types of arthritis (Badley, 1991), and increasing pressure on rheumatological services (Meenan, 1991; Symmons *et al.*, 1991). These changes also mean that there is an increasing number of people for whom a large part of everyday life is taken up with the process of learning to live with disease and its consequences. The third reason for the growing importance of understanding lay experiences relates to changes in society. There are many ways in which the power, prestige and status of medicine have been diminished over the last 20 years or so and a large number of challenges to medicine can now be seen to exist (Gabe *et al.*, 1994). Lay people are less convinced than they once were that doctors have all the answers to health problems, and are more prepared to say so (Popay and Williams, 1994). These long-term changes in culture and society have been fostered by policy changes related to governmental concern with the costs of health and social care.

When lay experiences of arthritis are seen against the background of these changes it becomes clear that the lay view has to be fully incorporated in our approaches to the therapeutic process. In understanding this process and how to respond to it, those engaged in treatment, rehabilitation and education cannot act as if they are writing on a 'blank sheet' (Donovan *et al.*, 1989).

WHAT DO WE MEAN BY EXPERIENCE?

In talking of the need to understand the experience of rheumatoid arthritis, or any other chronic illness, there are three broad areas that need to be considered (Bury, 1991): *coping*, *strategy* and *style*. Coping is a difficult concept to define because it has a variety of uses. Coping is a key concept in psychological medicine (Ray *et al.*, 1982), and it has been applied with considerable benefit in the field of rheumatic diseases (Newman and Revenson 1993; see Chapter 7 in this volume). Coping tends to be used to reflect, in part, the ways in which people understand the experience of illness: what they feel and think about it, how they understand it and explain it to themselves, how they attempt to tolerate its effects in relation to their perception of themselves and so on. This is a cognitive process which begins with the initial concern about symptoms, leading to the search for some kind of explanation for them, and continues throughout the process of adjustment (see also Leventhal *et al.*, 1984; Taylor, 1982).

Bury distinguishes this cognitive process from 'strategy', which relates to action. Coping efforts or strategies reflect the way in which people attempt to manage on a day-to-day basis with the consequences of chronic disease in their lives (see Chapter 7). This involves considering the illness in terms of the situation in which someone finds him or herself. While RA itself involves symptoms which need to be managed and coped with, the disadvantages which people experience in their daily lives may have less to do with the direct effects of the disease and more to do with the interaction between the individual and the social and physical world. In this area we are primarily concerned with the experience of illness in terms of its disabling, personal and social consequences for the individual – the experience of disability and handicap.

The third area is sometimes referred to as 'style' of adjustment (Bury, 1991; Radley, 1989). This refers primarily to the symbolic dimension, and involves examining the ways in which people handle the business of interaction, and how they present various features of their illness and their treatment regimen. In this area of illness experience the focus is on the 'cultural repertoires' that people can deploy in presenting the problem of, say, altered physical appearance or deteriorating social circumstances. In a sense, the style of adaptation involves attention to both aspects of the meaning of illness – its significance in the sense of how the individual integrates it into a life in a certain sort of culture and society – and its consequences in the sense of how the individual represents the experience to others in the course of daily life.

These three aspects of the experience of chronic illness – coping, strategy and style – are obviously closely interconnected within the life of any one individual. They cannot be treated separately within the therapeutic process, but in order to understand the complexity of what is sometimes referred to globally as the 'patient's point of view', and the success or otherwise with which people adapt or adjust to chronic illness, it is important to recognise the different processes to which they refer.

From the point of view of someone with arthritis there are a number of aspects to coping. The first is learning to tolerate the unpredictability in the symptoms; the second is developing explanations for what has happened; the third is establishing a sense of coherence through the reconstruction of one's understanding of the place of illness in life so as to maintain a belief in the meaning and value of one's life in spite of the symptoms and their effects (Taylor, 1982).

THE EXPERIENCE OF UNCERTAINTY

Uncertainty is part of everyday life. However, it has been clearly documented that the process of living with RA exacerbates uncertainty in a variety of ways (Wiener, 1975; Bury, 1982). This perspective is important because it makes us look at the illness as something that is similar to other experiences in life. The onset of chronic illness disrupts and constrains existing routines while simultaneously requiring the development of new routines in order to protect individuals from the worst effects of uncertainty. Uncertainty is something that is simultaneously psychological and social, cognitive and material, and therefore relates to coping.

For someone who develops RA, the early stages of the illness are fraught with uncertainty. While there are cases where RA begins suddenly, with the person going from well to ill within a very short time, in the vast majority of cases the onset is insidious, with the symptoms being present for months or even years before they are finally diagnosed or give rise to manifest disability (Locker, 1983). For people who develop the symptoms that eventually come to be diagnosed as RA, it is often very difficult to know whether something is 'really' going wrong; even when the person is convinced something is going wrong it is often difficult to convince others, both relatives and professionals, that this is the case. The phase of pre-diagnostic uncertainty can last for a considerable period. A woman woke up one night with pain in one arm and went through successive diagnoses of 'sprain', 'a bit of rheumatism', until RA was finally diagnosed 12 months later.

Before diagnosis

The prime source of uncertainty in the early stages lies in the disease itself. As RA symptoms include pain, joint stiffness and discomfort, and more generalised fatigue, individuals may find themselves vaguely aware that they cannot perform their everyday tasks as easily as they did. The process of coming to terms with these symptoms, and making some sense of them, is far from straightforward (Williams and Wood, 1987). For people who have experienced only acute illness episodes, where they are ill and then well again, symptoms that appear and disappear are difficult to understand (Leventhal *et al.*, 1984). For the person who develops RA difficulties arise with regard to normal understanding of bodily processes. 'It was just my knee . . .', one man reported, '. . . it just blew up for no reason. It wasn't painful to start with, just swollen. . . . It was a funny shape and I thought "what's going on here?" '

In the early stages of RA, therefore, there is often considerable confusion about whether real illness is present, and about the appropriate action to take. The ability to place symptoms within some pre-existing frame of reference is undermined (Leventhal *et al.*, 1984). Even something as apparently incontrovertible as pain is surrounded by uncertainty, and the pain varies in its intensity, duration and location in the various joints of the body. The pain moves or 'travels' as one respondent put it, to different sites in the body. Pain may appear in one joint only to be in a different joint the following day, and sometimes different kinds of pain co-exist – specific pains in one or two joints may be compounded by an overall aching. The symptoms are inconsistent both within an individual's experience over time, and between different people with the same diagnosis.

The experience of uncertainty, however, does not exist in some kind of vacuum. The individual's response to bodily disorder and the way in which it is coped with depends to some extent on background understanding and experiences (Bury, 1988). For example, one woman in her thirties who was a trained nurse, and who had a sister and an aunt who were severely disabled as a result of RA, was not surprisingly disturbed by the onset of joint pain in herself. She went through a period of considerable pre-diagnostic uncertainty until she was taken into hospital and put through a series of tests:

> They admitted me and I had a remission in hospital. They kept me in for a week and I had no sign at all. They took blood tests and there was nothing in my blood, and they came round and said to me: 'Well we've found out that there's nothing wrong with you.' Then, I'll never forget it, this doctor said to me: 'You're a nurse, your sister's got this disease, your auntie's got this disease, you're thinking about it too much. We all have aches and pains you know.' I felt terrible. I came out of there with my tail between my legs and I came home.

Descriptions of being defined as a malingerer or hypochondriac are not uncommon amongst people in the early stages of many chronic diseases (Anderson and Bury, 1988). In this woman's case, it was not until several months later, after it became almost impossible for her to care for herself and her young daughter, that she was readmitted to hospital and a diagnosis of RA was made. In the intervening period, she had visited several doctors and had become convinced that it must be 'all in the mind'.

The threat posed by these often vague symptoms may be compounded by the sometimes disbelieving response of close friends and relatives (Bury and Wood, 1978). For example:

> I think my mum was the worst. She kept saying, It's all in the mind. She got my husband believing the same things, and of course I thought I was going mental at the time.

The uncertainty at this stage primarily affects cognition. The validity of people's own interpretations of what is happening to them is open to question from all sides: from relatives and friends, from professionals, and from themselves.

After diagnosis

The way in which the quality of the uncertainty changes once a diagnosis has been made is something that has been noted in relation to RA and other chronic diseases. In one study of people with multiple sclerosis, for example, respondents described the pronouncement of the diagnosis as the cause of relief rather than horror (Stewart and Sullivan, 1982). The woman referred to above who had difficulty in convincing her mother and husband also remarked that although she did not feel glad that she had arthritis, she did feel relieved that she 'could say there was *something* I was moaning about'. At last there is an illness label (Leventhal *et al.*, 1984), something against which to place the many troubling circumstances which they had difficulty understanding, and which had been a source of embarrassment: in our society someone who falls over has either tripped or they are drunk.

Apart from the pain, the defining characteristic of a chronic disease such as RA is its unpredictability. While the diagnosis of RA removes one dimension of uncertainty, there is then the problem of how to respond to symptoms that are literally there one day and gone the next. Some individuals come to doubt the original diagnosis when they experience a long remission, only to be knocked back again when the symptoms reappear. While the unpredictability of RA can be described as something separate from the kind of life the person leads, the nature of the unpredictability is most apparent in looking at the relationships between bodily symptoms and the person's life. As Wiener has argued, people with RA are faced with having to accommodate themselves to an unpredictable body and to accept its dictates, while continuing to respond to the demands and requirements of daily life. Uncertainty and the strategies for coping with it emerge primarily from the interaction between these competing imperatives (Wiener, 1975).

Once diagnosed, other kinds of uncertainty become part of the individual's life, and the lives of those close to them. These uncertainties have a variety of implications for coping and for the valued 'style of life' that someone is able to sustain in response to the consequences and significance of RA. The first kind of uncertainty arises out of the questions 'why me?' and 'why now?', which relate to the problem of cause; the second relates to the anxiety raised by the question: 'what will happen to me?' which concerns the problem of outcome. Questions about the trajectory and the likely outcome are central (Locker, 1983), and of growing importance within health services. However, prior to that, analytically if not experientially, is the question of how people make sense of the development of RA in their lives.

LAY BELIEFS ABOUT ARTHRITIS

Lay or common-sense beliefs about illness have become the subject of considerable interest in a number of social sciences, including anthropology (Kleinman, 1988), sociology (Calnan, 1987; Fitzpatrick, 1989) and psychology (Leventhal *et al.*, 1984; Murray, 1990), and there have been suggestions of ways of integrating these (Landrine and Klonoff, 1992). They have also been increasingly related to aspects of patient management in clinical medicine (Wright and Hopkins, 1977; Chalmers, 1984). Work in this area has indicated how lay beliefs about illness are constituents of belief systems, and these belief systems are shaped by the culture and society of which they are a part.

Lay perspectives on the causes of arthritis

In being culturally shaped, the content and structure of lay beliefs exhibit considerable variation. In almost all studies, however, the issue of the cause of the illness is prominent. In one important study, Blaxter (1983) interviewed a sample of middle-aged women from working-class backgrounds with regard to their general ideas about health and illness. The issue of the cause of the illness was mentioned in 74 per cent of the examples. Blaxter noted how important it was for these women to be able to connect together various events in their lives, including the onset of illness. Other studies have noted similar variations and have gone on to try to group beliefs in terms of whether they refer to factors inside or outside individual control (Foster, 1976; Pill and Stott, 1982). Chrisman (1977) has noted the way in which 'folk ideas' appear to represent different modes of thought or 'logics': logics of degeneration, mechanical failure, imbalance and invasion.

There are a small number of studies that have addressed this issue in relation to arthritis. In one of the earliest, looking at beliefs about osteoarthrosis, Elder noted, 'The cause of arthritis symptoms . . . is unknown or, at best, controversial, and as a consequence official communications concerning it are limited. Thus a fertile field exists for the development of ideas derived from empirical experience and non-scientific beliefs about bodily functioning' (1973: 29). More than 20 years later the causes of arthritis symptoms remain obscure (see Chapter 2). Whether the problem is seen as one of inadequate scientific knowledge, inadequate translation of the knowledge that exists into lay terms, or a difference in the nature of the understanding required by doctors and patients, the process of making sense of symptoms described by Elder is of continuing relevance.

The focus of Elder's study of 180 people with osteoarthritis (OA) was the relationship between social class background and lay explanations for the aetiology of the illness. OA has traditionally been thought of in rather unproblematic terms as something which people get ineluctably as they age, as a consequence of wear and tear on the joints. In more recent years, the origin and pathogenesis of OA have been recognised as being less straightforward than they were once thought to be. The broad conclusions of this study were that those in higher social classes were more likely to attribute their symptoms to ageing, heredity, or to state that the cause was unknown, whereas those in lower social classes were more likely to stress the impact of the environment, including cold, damp, and adverse working conditions. Overall, Elder grouped respondents' causal explanations into eight categories: ageing, climate, exposure to the elements, working conditions, injuries, heredity, psychological distress and 'don't know'. In line with conventional clinical knowledge about OA, the most popular lay explanation was 'ageing', with 58 per cent of the sample believing that their symptoms were caused, at least in part, by the ageing process.

In another paper Gray (1983) looked at variations in beliefs about joint disease in general. The research population was 104 'arthritis sufferers', some of whom were contacted through a rheumatology clinic, and others picked up by their responses in a health-needs survey. This study therefore involved a group of people who were much more loosely 'arthritis and rheumatism sufferers', some diagnosed, some undiagnosed, although some of the respondents did use more specific terms such as 'osteoarthritis' and, less commonly, 'rheumatoid arthritis'. A similar diversity of aetiological beliefs was found in this study to that found in Elder's. Ideas about the cause of arthritis and rheumatism were divided into five categories: orthodox aetiological beliefs, heredity or ageing, hard work or over-use, uninformed lack of knowledge, and other unorthodox. Orthodox beliefs were most frequent but, overall, around three-quarters of the responses fell into categories other than that of orthodox beliefs. The categorisation of responses to questions about aetiology was complicated by the fact that respondents had different diagnoses. Therefore, the responses were assigned to categories on the basis of their appropriateness with respect to the illness from which the person claimed to be suffering. For example, those who attributed their osteoarthritis to the secondary effects of trauma had their responses allocated to the 'orthodox belief' category, whereas someone who attributed his or her 'gout' to the same cause was placed in the 'other unorthodox' category.

These studies demonstrate that lay beliefs about arthritis are many and varied. However, most of this work does little more than describe the associations that exist in people's minds between their arthritis and other things in their lives. The work of Williams and his colleagues, looking specifically and directly at lay beliefs about RA, attempts both to describe these simple associations and to explain their logic and purpose, and, as such, will be described in some detail (Williams, 1984, 1986; Williams and Wood, 1986). This work is based upon in-depth interviews with a small number of people who had been diagnosed with RA for at least 5 years. Using semi-structured interviews with an almost entirely open mode of questioning, all 29 respondents (18 women and 11 men) offered some kind of explanation for the cause of their arthritis. The wide variety of factors mentioned by respondents is shown in Table 3.1.

The most frequently mentioned factors related to stress/life crisis and heredity/genes, closely followed by physical trauma. The stress category included such features of life as specific losses through losing one's job or bereavement, as well as long-term,

Table 3.1 Rank order of causal categories amongst respondents

Category	*No. of respondents*
Stress/life crisis	12
Heredity/genes	11
Physical trauma	9
Occupation	7
Environment (including climate)	6
Virus/germs	5
Previous illness	3
Ageing	3
Personality type	3
Wear and tear	2
Divine influence	2
Don't know	2

Source: Williams (1986)

less dramatic strains imposed by problems at work or at home. Physical trauma was a difficult category to construct, and covered a heterogeneity of factors including fairly simple phenomena such as falls and knocks, as well as more complex and culturally significant events such as a hospital operation or miscarriage. Any taxonomy is problematic, and the assignment of particular factors to more general categories depends a great deal on taking account of the context in which the event was discussed. This kind of experiential knowledge can really only be gained through the use of relatively unstructured methods of data collection.

Although the causal categories are exhaustive, they are not necessarily exclusive, and one of the more important features of this work is that it went on to examine the *combinations* of explanations that respondents provided. This analysis revealed a complexity that contradicts the prevalent idea amongst health care professionals that lay ideas are simple or basic. Only five patients cited a single factor to explain their arthritis, and even these single factors varied in the complexity of the meaning that could be attributed to them. For example, the single factor might be 'a fall' or 'God'. More common was a belief in arthritis as linked to stress, overlapping with and including identification of the role that personality played in determining the degree to which the particular individual was vulnerable to the effects of those stressful circumstances. Another example might be where the respondent attributed the onset of arthritis to a knock sustained while at work, and went on to locate this incident within an analysis of work in which such incidents are part of everyday risk. However, patients' perspectives on the cause of their arthritis were often much more complex than these examples. Two-factor explanations were most common, but many respondents cited three or more factors as having had some bearing on the onset of their disease.

The most significant aspect of these causal beliefs which does not emerge from a simple listing of them, was the way in which multiple factors were accounted for and 'weighted' in any one person's experience. For example, where factors relating to occupation and a virus were both given particular emphasis, this was because the individual identified their occupation as having made them vulnerable to symptoms, and a virus was seen as playing a triggering or precipitant role. This work confirms the findings of the earlier studies, and also shows in more detail how complicated beliefs can be. In some cases these beliefs amounted to formal 'models' which drew together the impact of a large number of factors existing over a long period. These studies of arthritis show us that lay beliefs are many and varied, and that they are logically consistent and coherent. However, they also show us other qualities of lay beliefs which represent a form of knowledge that is different in kind from that used in and applied by medicine (Williams, 1984; Williams and Wood, 1986; Radley, 1993).

Lay knowledge and narrative reconstruction

While medical explanations for diseases are related to a body of formal scientific knowledge, patients' views are woven out of the threads of their experiences. These threads may include a strand of formal medical knowledge, taken from books or encounters with health professionals, but this strand is likely to be no more important than the information derived from other sources – friends, fellow sufferers, popular magazines and television programmes. What distinguishes some of the recent work on lay beliefs is its attempt to explain *why* these beliefs exist and take the forms they do. It is partly related to the vacuum of information about many diseases, including RA, but also involves the kind of information required by lay people and what that information is needed for.

In a carefully designed study, Linn *et al.* (1982) examined cancer patients' beliefs about the causes of their disorder, and compared these with those of a matched comparison group of patients with non-cancer diagnoses. What was most revealing was the researchers' aside that cancer patients seemed to be less certain in their identification and attribution of causal factors than the non-cancer patients. They speculate that this may be due to the complexity of the sufferers' awareness of causes, and that 'the closer he comes to dealing with the disease, the less clear-cut and more complex the explanations may become' (Linn *et al.*, 1982: 838).

This important insight casts doubt upon the validity of a simple division between exogenous and endogenous factors within lay beliefs. In both this study of cancer patients and the arthritis studies cited earlier, what is striking is the extent to which the most common causal categories either define the onset of disease in terms of external features of the world or in terms of features that are internal or relational, but largely outside the simple control of the individual. Thus, four out of the eleven categories in Linn *et al.*'s study are indicative of implacable and immutable externality and uncontrollability – inheritance, work, environment and God's will. The last of these could be interpreted as implying a degree of personal responsibility, but not necessarily so; and the category of 'work' has only a limited amount of choice attached to it. Similarly, in Elder's (1973) work on OA, the sense conveyed by the beliefs she describes is of the inevitability of the disease as an outcome of living in the kind of world we do.

The key point to be made about the illness beliefs amongst those who are ill is that they are complex and uncertain. This may be due in part to levels of formal knowledge, but what is more important is the meaning and purpose that the beliefs have for the individuals concerned (Herzlich and Pierret, 1985). For the non-cancer patients the problem posed was a relatively academic exercise. For the cancer patients it was an invitation to reflect on the meaning and purpose of their lives. For people asked to explain the aetiology of their own serious illness, particularly where there are strong cultural associations with death or with life in a wheelchair, the explanations are likely to have more nuances because they are also interpretations of the meaning of their own life and the lives of those close to them, and justifications of the way they have lived their lives.

It is clear that lay beliefs about illness are more than simple descriptors of a presumed causal process. They may also be seen as interpretations people use to reestablish some kind of cognitive order (Locker, 1981) in the face of the 'biographical disruption' (Bury 1982) chronic illness entails. In this sense, lay beliefs can be seen as an attempt to develop causal models to explain the onset and course of disease, and as narrative reconstructions of the relationship between the experience of illness and the person's autobiographical understanding of his or her own life (Williams, 1984; Williams and Wood, 1986; Kelly, 1986). Lay beliefs are part of an attempt to cope with a life that has been undermined by illness (Williams, 1986). The purpose of an individual's thinking, in these terms, is not primarily to develop a 'scientific' model of cause and effect, but to reconstruct a meaningful narrative out of the changes that have upset the meanings and purposes of the life.

The following extract from a lengthy interview with a 68-year-old man who had had RA for 20 years or more can serve as an illustration. He introduced this memory of war into the middle of a passage discussing what caused his RA:

> I went to North Africa, Italy, Austria, through and home. But we was getting drowned through the night, in Italy and Africa mostly, at Christmas time. We was going to make a big push at Christmas, but the weather was so bad that they cancelled it, and we was up to our knees in mud. In Italy there were weeks when I never wore a pair of socks, it was a waste of time. We was on this brow here and you couldn't stand up during the day. We dug little slits and you was in that slit all day lying in the sun, can't move, and at night it's throwing it down on you . . . and then they wonder why you're like this!
>
> (Williams and Wood, 1986: 1436)

Contained within this extract is something much more than an explanation of why he had developed RA. It is more an answer to the question: 'How have I come to be like this?', or 'Why has this happened to me, and why now?' It is both an attempt to explain the causes of the disease and to cope with the consequences of illness by placing it within a meaningful narrative.

Other people may refer to the stresses of personal relationships and family life and weave the cause of their arthritis into a narrative unfolding around those themes. A middle-class woman in her fifties said of the causes of her RA:

> I'm quite certain that it was stress that precipitated this. Not simply the stress of events that happened but the stress of

> suppressing myself while I was a mother and wife; not 'women's libby', but there comes a time in your life when you think, you know, 'where have I got to? There's nothing left of me'.
> (Williams, 1984: 188)

These lay beliefs can be read, in a 'quasi-scientific' mode, as attempts to construct causal models to explain the onset of RA. In their more complex forms these link together a number of factors over time to explain an event. At this level, the explanations are attempts to understand the complexities of a disease that is inadequately understood within biomedicine. However, in order to understand why people hold to these beliefs in spite of alternative information from experts they need to be seen as narrative reconstructions of a person's life with illness. In this 'biographical mode' they represent an attempt to find some kind of meaning and 'sense of coherence' (Antonovsky, 1979; Taylor, 1982). They are 'biographical body conceptions' which link subjective experience to daily life across the life-course (Corbin and Strauss, 1988).

LIVING DAY TO DAY

The process of coping with the effects of RA on identity and outlook is one important aspect of the experience. In the preceding sections we have looked at the meaning of RA in terms of its significance for the individuals concerned. Alongside this continual process of constructing and reconstructing identity in the face of the disruption of chronic arthritis, the individual is confronted with the need to develop strategies for coping with the consequences of arthritis day to day (Bury, 1991). Pain, stiffness and fatigue interfere in incalculable ways with the conduct of daily activities; both 'simple' activities such as going to the toilet, and more complex activities involving relationships with others. Whether simple or complex, many of these activities are so mundane that they are taken for granted until illness and disablement interfere (Locker, 1983).

Activities of daily living

Because of the taken-for-granted nature of such activities as washing and dressing, getting up from a chair or walking across a room, it is sometimes difficult for people to convey a sense of the limitations they confront. RA typically develops slowly, and in the early stages of the disease a person may look quite normal. Locker's (1983) respondents referred to the way in which it was the 'little things' that made them frustrated and aware of the fact that they had disabilities. At the level of individual activities and their constituent tasks, therefore, the things that are normally taken for granted become self-conscious and a matter for deliberation:

> Last night I thought it's time to put that hot water bottle in. Well, I couldn't get the top out could I . . . so I thought there must be a way . . . so I put a screwdriver through the top and turned it round. . . . Alright, it just needs a bit of thought and patience.
>
> (Williams, 1984: 287)

For people with RA the consequences manifest themselves in relation to almost all areas of daily life: sleep and rest, ambulation and body transfer, washing and bathing, dressing, mobility and 'housework' (Locker, 1983). It is only when it becomes difficult or impossible to do these things that people realise how significant they are. As Locker writes, 'mundane activities are important simply because they are mundane . . . a constant reminder that the individual is less than he or she once was' (1983: 95).

Strategies have to be developed to deal with the disabilities in specific areas. This may involve getting others to help, doing it oneself but doing it differently, or finding a substitute for the activity that can no longer be done. For example, in relation to keeping oneself clean people start showering instead of bathing, then make adaptations to the bathroom in order to continue being able to bath, and later dispense with bathing or showering and have a wash down, or bathe when they visit relatives (Locker, 1983).

The impact of RA upon daily activities is mediated by a sense of what activities ought to be performed. People sometimes define themselves as 'doers' who can no longer do things. As one man put it: 'I'm just one of those people who likes to be doing things, you see. When you can't do . . . it just comes to a dead stop.' However, the extent to which a particular activity is problematic depends on the context in which it is performed (Locker, 1983). The inability to open a tin of food is no problem if you have never wanted or needed to do it, and there is somebody else there to do it for you. The experience of RA must be examined in relation to the context in which people live. It is this wider contextual aspect of chronic illness that is underplayed in most rehabilitation studies of activities of everyday life (Williams, 1987). The context will be considered in terms of three key dimensions: roles, relationships and routines.

The importance of social roles

Tasks and activities are organised in terms of social roles. Role is an important concept in which to understand daily life experiences because of the way in which it links the individual and society (Goffman, 1972). Activities are performed within social roles and it is in relation to roles that such tasks and activities have symbolic significance. The activities themselves may not seem particularly grand or important, but their place within a role may accord them enormous significance.

Take, for example, the tying of shoelaces, which involves a degree of manual dexterity that is a particular problem for many people with RA (Mason *et al.*, 1983). Sometimes it may be possible to make simple adaptations such as altering the type of footwear. However, when the person with RA is a mother, struggling to get her two children off to the school where the children are required to wear lace-up shoes, the social effects run deep. This may appear to be an artificial problem, easily solved, but one woman who gave her account of this experience told how devastated she had felt at the time. A simple activity like tying shoelaces may also be a vehicle through which a social role is enacted and a sense of identity confirmed. It is because of this that specific disabilities can have more general consequences for a person with RA. Where an activity is part of a caring role, the failure in this activity can have profound ramifications. (This is discussed more within the context of social support reciprocity in Chapter 8.)

A more clear-cut example of a situation in which the meaning of activities varies with social role is provided by the situation of some women with RA. The importance of activities associated with nurturing and homemaking such as shopping and cooking, depends on the position someone occupies in the domestic division of labour (Bury, 1985; Reisine *et al.*, 1987). Although men may share in some of the domestic tasks, this role responsibility remains firmly with women (Oakley, 1985), even with wives who have RA (Revenson, 1994a, b). As one woman with RA put it:

> If I am trying to do something (in the kitchen) and I get frustrated, I'll be cursing and (my husband) says, 'Why do you try to do it? I'll do it for you if you ask me.' And I say: 'Well I shouldn't have to ask you.'
>
> (Williams, 1987: 99)

The nature of household roles and 'the family' has changed over the past 20 years, but for a woman living in a traditional nuclear family where the husband is the 'breadwinner' and she is the 'homemaker' the inability to prepare a meal can be a profoundly unsettling experience because it is a basic activity through which her social role is delineated. As one woman put it: 'You feel a bit incomplete, I suppose', while another explained:

> I've got a guilt complex. I don't feel the children and my husband should do so much of my work, I feel I should take a bigger part. He will cook a meal sometimes if I've been really bad and I feel really guilty.
>
> (Williams, 1987: 99)

It is not just a problem of the inability to perform certain activities, but the failure in the *performance* of social roles. Performance is an important term here because, according to the dictionary, it is both the accomplishment of an action and a ceremony. Cutting and peeling vegetables, cooking, putting food on the table and washing up can be seen both as discrete activities for which the symptoms of RA cause difficulties, and as parts of the ceremony of family life for many people.

These different levels of activity and role performance are important in understanding the kinds of strategies people develop for dealing with their difficulties. At the level of specific tasks, people with RA develop techniques for undertaking discrete activities, often using adaptations to help in this. But in terms of the overall performance, the problems can be tackled more holistically. Rather than struggling to find new ways of doing things, for example, it is sometimes possible to alter the overall division of labour and the expectations about who does what in the household. One woman, for example, offered her children payment for cleaning windows and doing the shopping. Another said: 'I can't lift pans with vegetables in. The kids empty the vegetable water and serve up everything, but I organize it. I say what we're going to buy and what we're going to eat.' By redefining her role in relation to the preparation of food as supervisory and managerial rather than operational, she managed to maintain a sense of competent involvement in the ongoing performance in spite of her disabilities.

The importance of roles persists beyond the household. Although many people with RA have to give up work, others try to develop ways of adapting to the demands of their work in relation to their symptoms. One man who worked as a painter and decorator described this kind of process:

> There were days when I couldn't really use a paintbrush in one hand. So I would get a piece of sandpaper and use the left hand and do a bit of sandpapering down for the next hour or so, ready for the next day . . . and I kept going!

The advice from a doctor to give up work, while sensible at one level, is often not practical. Non-adherence with treatment recommendations is often discussed as if it were an individual choice, but it may be quite unrelated to the structural realities of everyday life. One woman recognised how badly her RA was being affected by her continuing to work but said: 'it was necessity you see. My husband's only in a low wage bracket, and it did help pay the mortgage and keep things going properly here.' Moreover, even where it is economically feasible, a person may have such a profound symbolic investment in their work, and define themselves in terms of it, that to give up work would be difficult to contemplate.

Failure to perform certain tasks is a major aspect of the experience of RA. These failures and the strategies used to offset them often are important in themselves, but are particularly informative as they represent failures in the performance of social roles. Individuals evaluate their activity performance in terms of the extent to which they are enacting meaningful roles and performing them well. It has been implicit in what has been said so far that this performance has implications for relationships of interdependence with others, and it is to that we now turn.

Dependence in relationships

In the same way that activity restriction in RA can be fully understood only in relation to social roles, so dependence can be understood only in the context of the relationships between people in different social roles. At home and at work people exist in shifting relations of interdependence, and the relative autonomy of individuals within roles depends upon external factors such as the quality of local neighbourhoods and the state of the local and national economies.

The onset of RA disrupts normal patterns of interdependence. The severity of this disruption varies with the nature of the onset and the stability of the setting within which the person lives. One woman who had a severe and rapid onset of RA said:

> I just used to lie and shiver and couldn't move. Having got downstairs in the morning I used to spend most of the day wondering if my son and husband would get me back up there in the evening.
>
> (Williams 1987: 100)

Studies of the experience of RA indicate that 'dependence' gives rise to a great deal of anxiety and fear (Locker, 1983; Williams and Wood, 1988). In light of the characteristic pattern of remission and relapse in RA, heavy dependency such as that depicted by the woman above is unusual and occasional. While dependency in rehabilitation studies is normally discussed in terms of the inability to perform key tasks such as washing and cooking, the experience for the individual is one of having to rely on others to do things. Dependency is not so much an individual state but a quality of social relationships, and it is most often expressed as the fear of being a burden on others, particularly those close to the person with RA.

Dependency is generally described by people with RA as a process of giving up responsibility for doing certain things – whether they are self-care activities or wider roles – to others. As one man said to his wife in the context of an interview about his RA: 'It was upsetting me because you were having to do a lot of things I should have done.' The concern was both a loss of ownership and control over activities and the feeling that this loss of autonomy imposed illegitimate burdens on others. Very often people with RA do not want help unless they ask for it, but they are also reluctant to ask. As one woman put it: 'It's alright me saying I've got relations – my sister will come and tidy up and everything for me – but they have their own lives to live, they have their own families to see to.' The experience of dependence was characterised by always having to ask other people to do certain things, and having to wait for other people to be around to help. One woman, referring to her husband, said:

> I think he gets a bit fed up sometimes. He comes home a bit tired and I say, 'Oh could you just do so and so', and he rolls his eyes and I think, 'Oh I shouldn't have to ask him that.' You know, sometimes you don't want to ask anything of anybody really.

The essentially relational quality of dependence (and independence) is seen in terms such as 'being a burden to others', and 'not wanting to interfere with' the lives of others. Dependence inherently has to do with social relationships, and discomfort comes both from the sense of depersonalisation that can follow from having things done for you, and from the feeling that certain tacit moral rules about what can be expected of others are being infringed. Drawing too freely upon the time of other family members is seen, literally, as taking liberties.

For people with RA, as with other chronic illnesses, this is felt more strongly in some relationships than others, and is related to the degree to which expected patterns of caring and being cared for are reversed, for example, in situations where a woman in her forties needs the support of an elderly mother. One 30-year-old woman and her baby daughter were both being looked after by her mother who was in her mid-sixties. This caused a double burden of guilt and anxiety – failing to discharge her own duties to her baby and imposing unfair demands on her mother. The feeling of concern about dependence in relationships for people with RA is felt most acutely in their relationships with their children: 'I don't want to be a burden to my family, that's the main thing. I'd hate to think that because I've seen so many people be a burden to their children and I think it's most unfair.'

Although people with RA may talk with horror of becoming dependent, the reality of daily life for most is a gradual and subtle alteration in their relationships with a range of informal and formal networks. RA is a process, not a state. For some people, having struggled to do everything for themselves, there comes a point where they accept a change in their relationships: 'It would be about the middle of when I was ill that I began to settle for them (the family) to do things for me.' Having 'rebelled' against the situation at first this woman eventually reached some kind of settlement with herself and the situation she was in. However, this settlement is always provisional. Living with chronic illness involves continual adjustment to changing aspects of disease, alterations in the domestic milieux, the varying availability of benefits and services, and changes in the wider economic and social situation.

Although this discussion of dependence in relationships has centred on the domestic milieu, this milieu and the relationships within it are underpinned by the wider situation. People with RA will often turn to the resources outside of the home in order to prevent problems of dependence on close relatives. For example, one woman, although having two sons living nearby, was helped in her bathing by the district nursing service. For her, dependence upon anyone was disliked, and she found her life transformed by a bath-seat: 'So I got one of those and it's smashing. With that I've got independence. I can go up and have a bath when I want, you know, without asking anybody.' The provision of simple aids and adaptations can transform personal and social relationships (Locker, 1983), and although dependence upon an object can be uncomfortable it has fewer connotations than dependence on other people, be they relatives or statutory services. While dependence upon a mechanical aid can be upsetting because it exists as a constant reminder of disablement, it avoids the complications of reciprocity and indebtedness (Williams, 1993).

SUMMARY

The effects of RA on individuals' experiences are profound. In this chapter we have tried to show the extent of these effects, as much as possible through the words of people with arthritis themselves. This chapter has explored the experience of chronic illness in terms of its meaning: its significance and its consequences. We have tried to convey a sense of the more general social experience and impact of RA and not simply the experience of symptoms. In doing so we hope to have drawn attention to those features that RA shares with other chronic illnesses: it is because RA is a *chronic* illness that it undermines identity and disrupts roles and relationships. We all suffer pain from time to time; we all have occasional experiences of frustration at finding that our bodies do not perform at the level we would expect, and we suddenly realise we are getting older; we all go through periods of looking back on our lives and being dismayed at how things have changed; we all sometimes feel too tired to go to the party. These are the everyday biographical disruptions to which people with RA are exposed. While it is difficult to imagine a society or a situation in which RA would not be an unpleasant and distressing experience, it is possible to imagine a situation in which people's sense of their own significance could be supported, and the social consequences of their disabilities could be cushioned. However, this would involve seeing people as a whole and acknowledging the extent to which society limits the adjustments people can make.

Chapter 4

Pain and stiffness

INTRODUCTION

Pain and stiffness are the cardinal symptoms of RA. For most patients they shape the experience of living with RA and they affect disability in both the short and long-term. Aims of the management of arthritis are to 'minimise pain, disability, deformity and the social/psychological dysfunction which often accompany painful illness' (Lorig *et al.*, 1987: 208). Many studies provide supporting evidence to show that pain, stiffness and disability are major concerns for those with RA (Parker, Frank *et al.*, 1988). Deyo (1988) observes that people are more concerned about being free of pain and being able to perform their usual activities than about the results of their latest laboratory test. This is just as well, because the results from many of these tests are quite unreliable, as Deyo demonstrates. Such findings support the idea that self-report measures of pain and disability may be a better way of assessing quality of life. They not only save the physician's time, but also provide an indication of the priorities patients hold about their own treatment (Liang *et al.*, 1978).

However, Barnes and Mason (1975) point out that these 'outstanding symptoms . . . are often difficult to separate'. Duration of morning stiffness appears to be a useful marker of disease and if it lasts more than an hour, is deemed to be clinically significant. For the majority of people with RA, pain has an insidious rather than acute onset and in the early stages occurs during movement, but as disease activity increases, spontaneous pain at rest develops. Pain and stiffness are frequently preceded and accompanied by fatigue, weight-loss and feelings of ill-health (Huskisson & Hart, 1978).

In this chapter we will examine a variety of perspectives which assist understanding about how pain and stiffness are experienced by those with RA. First we examine some of the biological factors which are understood to generate pain and stiffness in RA patients then go on to look at the relationship of pain and stiffness to disability. In the third section some beliefs about the experience of pain are considered and finally we assess how pain and stiffness have been measured.

BIOLOGICAL ASPECTS OF PAIN AND STIFFNESS

In this section the mechanisms of pain and stiffness will be described. Inflammation of the synovial membrane (which creates the lubricating fluid for the joint) is represented by warmth, redness, tenderness or swelling (Fries, 1979). These changes can potentially affect any of the 187 synovial joints in the body. At its most severe, RA may include painful teno-synovitis, nodules, cysts and muscle and ligament wasting. Most pain in RA arises from pressure on the joint capsule and adjacent ligaments. Increased synovial fluid in the joint cavity and proliferation of the inflamed synovial tissues causes pain by distension, stretching and twisting of the capsule. While some areas of the joint are devoid of nerve endings and so are insensitive to inflammation, in sensitive areas several types of mechano-receptors have been identified as relevant to the generation of pain in arthritis. These sensory organs are Ruffini-like receptors in the articular capsule, Golgi tendon organs in the ligaments and Pacinian-style corpuscles in the capsule. Particularly important are the free nerve endings commonly found in joints.

These receptors are innervated by thinly myelinated and unmyelinated afferent nerve fibres which connect them to the central nervous system (CNS). Stimulation studies have found that some units are excited by innocuous movements of the knee joint and some monotonically respond to stimulation across the range from innocuous to noxious. There are also units which only appear to respond to noxious joint movement and others which under normal circumstances cannot be activated by any joint movement (see Campbell *et al.*, 1989 for a review). While these conclusions largely rely on investigations of cats so that the generalisation of results is questionable, at the same time they do provide insight into why inflamed tissues are highly sensitive to even gentle pressure and the slightest movement.

Most recently pain in arthritis has been investigated using experimentally induced arthritis (EA) in laboratory rats. Dubner (1989) provides a valuable review of the different methods of pain assessment tested in the pursuit of a reliable and valid animal model of arthritis. For instance, injection of an adjuvant such as a suspension of mycobacterium butyricum intradermally induces soft tissue swelling, a decrease in bone density (osteoporosis), cartilage loss and bone erosions. Adjuvant arthritis in rats is associated with chronic pain; they show increased sensitivity to paw pressure, lose weight, have disrupted sleep patterns, decrease their activity, hyperventilate and are irritated and hyperactive when handled. Sectioning the appropriate ascending CNS nerves partially relieves this pain and such rats show preferences for solutions containing non-steroidal anti-inflammatory drugs (NSAIDs) and low dose opiates. These drugs have had considerable clinical successes in reducing pain and inflammation in humans (Fitzgerald, 1989).

The gate control theory of pain originated by Melzack and Wall (1965, 1982) and Wall and Melzack (1989) is still, after 25 years, the major working theory. In a simplified form, it is theorised that sustained activity in unmyelinated C-fibres can lower thresholds at the spinal level by moderating the effect of incoming impulses from myelinated and larger A-fibres. A 'gating' mechanism in the hypothetical transmission of T-cells in the dorsal horns of the spinal cord, which is influenced by descending information from the brain – especially the thalamus – permits or prevents inputs from the periphery and internal organs from being experienced as pain. While the exact transmission cells have yet to be identified, there is considerable empirical support for a good approximation to this idea. There is gathering evidence that with repeated stimulation, plastic changes take place in the RNA of hypersensitive neurons so that eventually the 'gate' is held irreversibly open for those in chronic pain.

Studies of the thalamus and somato-sensory cortex show that, in arthritic conditions, some cells have an unusual and abnormally large response to joint stimulation, indicating long-term changes in the way impulses are processed. Looking at the response of rat somato-sensory cells to stimulation following prior injection of Freund's adjuvant, Guildbaud *et al.* (1989) report that while few neurons are activated by strong mechanical stimulation, around 50 per cent of cells in this region are activated by light pressure and brushing. The ventrobasal neurons of the thalamus also behave rather differently from other thalamic nuclei cells which suggests that they may be implicated in processing the sensory-discriminative aspects of pain (see Randlich, 1993). There is gathering evidence that at least some of these changes in the CNS are due to chronic pain (Guilbaud *et al.*, 1989). Work on the plasticity of neurons is important in the understanding and treatment of chronically painful diseases like RA. Such a mechanism gives some insight into why chronic pain is so resistant to treatment.

Stiffness is a much-neglected area of research. If pain is a difficult symptom to study then what about the elusive qualities of stiffness? Here some conceptual work is needed on whether stiffness is just one of the many qualities of pain or whether it is a discrete symptom which needs separate investigation in its own right and perhaps with different methodologies. The sensation of stiffness results from receptors in the joint capsule and ligaments and from the muscles and tendons which supply these joints. Helliwell and Wright (1991) draw out similarities between the mechanisms of pain and stiffness which may be elucidated by studying the neurophysiological changes believed to take place at a spinal level in the dorsal horns. Pain arising from chronic inflammation in joints lowers perception thresholds to mechanical stimuli as a result of synaptic influences at this spinal level. Helliwell and Wright have questioned whether perceptions of movement and vibration affect thresholds at different stages of arthritic disease.

This direct application of the gate control theory to explain both symptoms of stiffness and pain is welcome, because in many discussions of pain in arthritis this theory does not appear to have visibly influenced thinking in research, clinical practice or treatment over 25 years (e.g. Grennan and Jayson, 1989). While imperfect, the gate control theory does provide a reasoned neurophysiological and anatomical explanation for why there are patients attending rheumatology clinics who report pain in the joints but have no ostensible organic damage, such as in the case of sero-negative rheumatoid arthritis. Conversely, it explains why some people with the organic signs of RA in their joints and blood stream never complain of pain. The answer hinges not only on the gating mechanism in the dorsal horns but also on the descending controls – psychological and physiological – which are exerted by the brain on this process (Melzack and Wall, 1982; Wall and Melzack, 1989). It is the first theory of pain to formally integrate the wide range of psychological mechanisms which contribute to the experience and reporting of pain.

The nervous system does more than just signal pain from affected joints in RA (Fitzgerald 1989). Recent work by Levine's group (see Fitzgerald, 1989) has shown that primary afferent nociceptors are innervated by a branch of the sympathetic nervous system (SNS) and so contribute to the production of inflammation in a process of neurogenic inflammation. The results of sympathectomy and the use of beta-adrenergic receptor blockers provide support for this view and hence 'offer real scope for treatment' (Fitzgerald, 1989). Fitzgerald reorientates thinking in this area by presenting a model to show how pain is a part of the disease process and not simply a result of it.

In addition to environmental triggers such as infections like rubella, hepatitis-B and slow-acting viruses, genetic factors have been linked with the specific immune response of arthritis and it seems likely that both genetic and environmental factors are major contributors to the pathogenesis of the disease (see Chapter 2). Pincus and Callahan (1986) observed that parents of RA patients died on average 4 years younger than parents of those with osteoarthritis (OA), so giving support to genetic theories. Rheumatoid factor has also been documented in the serum of healthy relatives. The prominence of DR4 in the genetic composition of northern Europeans, Caucasoids and Israeli Jews goes some way to explaining the uneven incidence of the disease internationally (Grennan and Jayson, 1989).

There is an increased likelihood of the presence of histocompatibility antigens DR4 and D4 in those with sero-positive RA and the more erosive forms of the disease. Those with such antigens may be more predisposed to having injuries of blood vessels in the synovium with inflammation thrombosis and antibody production. The immune complexes of these antibodies and antigens increase vascular permeability so creating an influx of serum proteins and cellular components. White blood cells absorb these immune complexes and it is at this point that damage to the delicate synovium (three cells thick) and cartilage occurs. With synovial hypertrophy, granulation tissue called a pannus is formed. This produces sufficient enzymes like prostaglandins and collaginase, to attack and destroy the bone and cartilage around the joint capsule. An aim of treatment is to block this self-destructive activity in a way that the body fails to do for itself. Not only does this result in the loss of cartilage and a reduction in joint space but also the creation of bony erosions at the joint margins (Grennan and Jayson, 1989).

There is gathering evidence to support a link between the immunological, psychological and disease activity aspects of the disease. Recent analysis of data from a cross-sectional study has shown that the immune activation measure of HLA-DR+ cells in peripheral blood and levels of perceived helplessness were significantly related to an index of disease activity, namely joint count. Furthermore, disease activity significantly influenced levels of depression, while depression in turn affected pain perception but not vice versa (Parker *et al.*, 1992). However, longitudinal data support the reverse case, namely that pain influences depression.

PAIN, STIFFNESS AND DISABILITY

Pain, stiffness and the accompanying disability of arthritis are costly at many levels. Meenan *et al.* (1981) found that those diagnosed with RA earned only 50 per cent of the income predicted for them, had they been in good health. To these economic costs can be added the personal costs of the experience of pain and suffering and indirect costs to the patient's family (Akehurst, 1992; see Chapter 3). But although RA can profoundly affect functioning, it is a fallacy that this disease is a 'passport to a wheelchair' (Barnes and Mason, 1975). Around a quarter of those who attend for treatment recover completely, a further quarter heal but have residual damage to the joints which does not interfere with activities such as working and 40 per cent have continual disease activity but are not bedridden. Contrary to the popular image of the disease, only 10 per cent are severely crippled (Jayson and Dixon, 1980).

The many ways in which RA affects work, income and the psychosocial aspects of life are well documented. Inevitably they are interlinked as income and psychosocial factors are affected by work disability (Meenan *et al.*, 1981). Yelin *et al.* (1980) observe that where arthritis is concerned, there appear to be variables other than the degree of impairment, which affect changes in the labour supply. Reviewing evidence for a model by Berkowitz and others which proposes that social factors may be more important than medical ones in determining whether or not people will become disabled, they showed evidence that this is particularly true for those with RA in the mid-range of disease severity.

Following a survey of 245 RA patients, Yelin *et al.* (1980) showed that the four best variables measuring the social characteristics of work which included being able to control the pace of work and being self-employed, had better explanatory power (1.8 times greater) than the four best medical items they tested. These features had over twice the predictive power of the four best demographic items and 2.7 times that of the four best personal resource items. The reason why those who are able to control their work and are self-employed are more likely to continue working is probably because they have greater flexibility in their work patterns. For instance they may be able to defer an early start in the morning to take account of their stiffness, can adjust the pace of work to their needs, leave work early or take time off to accommodate the pain and discomfort of a 'flare'. Results from longitudinal and cross-sectional studies confirm that to keep people with arthritis within the workforce, flexible working conditions are essential (Yelin, *et al.*, 1987).

Much has been written about the link between pain, disability and depression and about how these factors affect each other. In one longitudinal study lasting 6 months, pain proved to be a significant predictor of subsequent physical disability. However, although physical disability is often coupled with pain, no fixed and consistent relationship has been established between the amount of demonstrable disease and degree of subjective distress (Kazis *et al.*, 1983).

THE EXPERIENCE OF PAIN AND STIFFNESS

What is the image people have of arthritis and do they expect to have pain and stiffness as symptoms? A report from a British community survey of 503 people recorded that the public were 'unanimous' that arthritis is a very painful disease and not just another name for normal aches and pains (Badley and Wood, 1979). Expectations of pain, stiffness, tenderness and swelling in the joints were commonly reported by US telephone respondents randomly contacted by Price *et al.* (1983). Using a sample stratified by age, sex and social class, Elder (1973) identified those who acknowledged three symptoms of arthritis and included all those in the 45–64 age group who reported morning stiffness, which was widely accepted as a symptom of arthritis. The majority of respondents also reported one or both symptoms of pain or swelling. Out of 160 people interviewed she found that the term arthritis was used freely to describe persistent aches, pains and stiffness associated with joints. Of these, half had learned to label it arthritis from their physician, the rest from lay people, TV or 'just knowing' it was a problem of the joints. So while there was evidence to show that they were unable to distinguish RA from osteoarthritis, these studies show that the general public is quite realistic and fairly knowledgeable about arthritis symptoms.

But even though people's expectations about arthritis are reasonably accurate, this does not much reduce the burden of coping with the disease if it occurs. Some researchers have argued that while pain, stiffness and disability are in their own right difficult to cope with, uncertainty about whether they will be present, and if so, to what degree can be disquieting and highly disruptive (Bury, 1982). In a qualitative in-depth study of twenty-one patients, Wiener (1975) showed that uncertainty was a key issue and furthermore was one which 'accounted for most of the variation in the psychosocial problem of living with RA' (p. 98). The peaks and troughs of wellness and flares can be quite unpredictable. There is also considerable variation in the severity, progression and areas of joint involvement in the disease. Uncertainty about whether there will be any pain, swelling or stiffness, which area(s) will be involved, how intense any disability will be, whether the onset will be sudden or gradual, how long it will last and how often flares will occur (Wiener, 1975) can be profoundly disabling.

Uncertainty can be a particular problem in the early stages of the disease when patients want information (Baker, 1981). Yet establishing a diagnosis and prognosis is difficult and because of this, often delayed. In their instructions to clinicians dealing with rheumatoid arthritis patients, Huskisson and Hart (1978) implicitly acknowledge the importance of uncertainty as they list making a firm diagnosis the number one priority of treatment. When outcomes are uncertain patients may view a reluctance to provide information as evasiveness and interpret this as an unwillingness to give bad news. Furthermore, any such suspicions may dampen questioning at the very time when active self-help should be encouraged. In line with Fordyce's (1988) view about the management of low back pain, Baker says that advice to rest might plausibly be misinterpreted as 'take it easy'. Such misinterpreted directions could have long-term counterproductive effects of producing iatrogenic disability.

Unpredictability also affects mental health, predisposing patients to anxiety and depression. These in turn may produce increased perceptions of pain and pain behaviour as well as reductions in attempts to cope or perform activities of daily living (Bradley *et al.*, 1984). There is gathering evidence that perceived unpredictability and loss of control related to beliefs in chance happenings facilitate the development of helplessness in those with chronic back pain (Skevington, 1983). In a study of ninety-two patients with RA, Affleck, Tennen, Pfieffer and Fifield (1987) found that those who expressed more personal control over their symptoms and over the course of the disease saw their illness as more predictable and this reduced uncertainty. Further analysis showed that if patients believed they had personal control over their treatment, they were also more likely to have a positive mood and better psychosocial adjustment. But negative mood was related to beliefs that others, such as health care providers, were more in control of their symptoms, particularly for the severely ill. These findings concur with those from a large literature on the loci of control and health which generally confirms that perceived internal or personal control is conducive to being more mentally healthy.

THE MEASUREMENT OF PAIN AND STIFFNESS

While there are several methods which might be used in the measurement of pain in RA, in this section we will confine discussion to work on the language of pain. Gracely has commented: 'Accurate appraisal of the biochemical, neuronal and psychological mechanisms of pain depends heavily on the assessment of pain in human subjects. Man's unique verbal abilities open a window to private experience and only through such experience is pain defined' (quoted by McQuay, 1990). The use of these abilities to describe the pain of RA produces some interesting similes: 'like walking on stones' (Grennan and Jayson, 1989) and 'like being in a suit of armour which is too tight' (Skevington, 1991).

But how can pain best be assessed? There have been many proposals about how the language of pain might be usefully structured and categorised. One of these has been to collect systematic clinical information from patients about their pain. A comprehensive self-assessment form has been outlined by Monks and Taenzer (1983) for this purpose. Answering is speeded by the provision of checklists for those concerned about time constraints. A guide to interviewers documents sociodemographic information, supplementary questions and the items from the McGill Pain Questionnaire (see below). The final section provides scope for making observations and judgements about the patient's behaviour during the interview, their mood and other impressions. Through the thorough and detailed clinical record-keeping, information about particular pain-patient populations such as those with the rheumatic diseases, might be more easily compiled and compared over long periods within and between institutions.

A more structured approach to investigating pain and disability comes from the Pain Disability Index (PDI) whose properties have been tested psychometrically on 444 chronic pain patients (Tait *et al.*, 1990). Tait *et al.* confirmed construct validity by showing that high scorers on the PDI reported more psychological distress, more severe pain and more restricted activities than low scorers. Nine variables were particularly important in predicting their score, these were time spent in bed, psychosomatic symptoms, stopping activities because of pain, work states, pain duration, usual pain intensity, quality of life, pain extent and education. Further work is needed to establish whether this is a useful measure for managing pain in RA.

The Visual Analogue Scale (VAS) was developed with the aim of measuring arthritis pain (Huskisson, 1983). This simple linear bipolar scale has been widely used as a single measure of pain intensity as it is relatively easy to use and score. The 100mm line is marked and measured to indicate a dimension from, say, worst pain ever to no pain at all, although the labels may be varied. Gaston-Johansson and Gustafsson (1990) examined the pain recorded from using the VAS in 30 RA patients and compared it with the pain intensity they reported while using the Ritchie Articular Index (pain associated with joint pressure). They found the two to be highly correlated, suggesting that they measure the same disease component. Both measures also correlated well with income, sick days and amount of sickness compensation.

The VAS has been adapted to measure pain relief in rheumatology using the Visual Analogue of Pain Relief Scale (VAPRS). Here the scale is divided into twenty parts from complete relief to no relief. While the originators considered the lack of a baseline to be an advantage, other users have commented that it is misleading to assume that all patients start from the same baseline of pain (Langley and Sheppard, 1985). Langley and Sheppard claim that a Visual Analogue Pain Severity Scale (VAPSS) which ranged from no pain to unbearable or worst pain is less prone to bias than the VAPRS. At the same time it draws on experimental knowledge in psychophysics which shows that pain sufferers are capable of detecting twenty-one different levels of pain when performing difference judgements.

The McGill Pain Questionnaire (MPQ) has made a substantial difference to the conceptualisation and measurement of pain because it assesses seventy-eight qualities of pain rather than the single quantity or intensity of pain conventionally measured by the Visual Analogue Scale. Each quality is weighted on a five-point scale. Grouped into sensory, affective and evaluative pain descriptions, the accumulated weightings from these three subscales have some predictive power clinically. The MPQ was standardised on a wide range of chronic pain patients including a small group with RA and OA ($n = 16$) (Melzack, 1975). Melzack (1975) reported that the majority of these arthritis patients used words like aching, exhausting and rhythmic to describe their pain and more than a third mentioned gnawing, annoying and constant. As persistent gnawing in the fingers may mean arthritis, it is therefore not surprising that one aim is to use this method to earmark qualities of pain as an aid to diagnosis (Melzack & Wall, 1989). A recent short form of fifteen descriptors is available (SF–MPQ) (Melzack, 1987). However it is too early to say whether this short form will be useful in the assessment of RA patients. As in the long form, stiffness is not included as a pain quality and this seems to be a serious omission where discomfort in RA is a concern.

Using a sample of 135 classical or definite RA patients who completed the MPQ, Parker, Frank *et al.* (1988) found that the group reported moderate to mild pain which was present all the time for 69 per cent of patients. The mean weightings were 13.3

for sensory pain, 2.1 for affective pain and 1.9 for evaluative pain. A closer look at the words selected showed that over 40 per cent of the sample reported sharp, tender, tiring, throbbing and aching pain. When classified on standardised ratings of functional class (Steinbrocker *et al.*, 1949), patients from functional class III ('functional capacity quite limited') reported more pain on a VAS of pain intensity and that a greater area of their body was painful, than for those from classes I and II ('complete functional capacity; functional capacity adequate to conduct normal activities despite handicap of discomfort or limited mobility of one or more joints'). More importantly their results showed that medical variables like erythrocyte sedimentation rate (ESR), swelling and tenderness on the Ritchie Articular Index, grip strength, walking speed and morning stiffness were only able to account for a mere 3 per cent of the variance in pain scores. The sociodemographic factors of age and income were much better predictors.

The language of RA pain reported by Parker *et al.* largely concurs with that from other studies. Wagstaff *et al.* (1985) reported that thirty-one RAs with an average duration of 9 years' illness described their pain as throbbing and burning, but never as scalding, drilling or cutting. They found that in general, the punctate and thermal pain subgroups of descriptors best discriminated between samples of OA and RA patients and that RAs were most likely to select a heat factor. However Nehemkis *et al.* (1985) have questioned the ability of these adjectives to discriminate between OA and RA. Skevington (1979, 1986) found that burning, aching and nagging were indicated by RAs with all types of immunological condition, but that stabbing, hot and sharp were particularly likely to be used by those with a sero-negative illness.

The persistence of pain during rest is one sign that the disease is progressing and Papageorgiou and Badley (1989) have shown how important it is to look at descriptors chosen for both resting and moving states. Using a selection of MPQ pain adjectives most frequently used by RA patients, they asked 105 patients to choose and volunteer words that best described their pain and to complete a VAS of pain intensity at rest and on movement. All had pain on movement, but only eighty-five also had pain at rest. Those descriptions most frequently chosen overall were tiring (78 per cent), troublesome (71 per cent), miserable (70 per cent), exhausting (66 per cent) and annoying (59 per cent). They volunteered the words frustrating, depressing and demoralising.

However pain at rest was most likely to be described as throbbing or aching, whereas shooting and spreading better described pain on movement. Some differences were found in the words used to describe the pain of particular joints, for example tender and sore tended to be used to describe rest pain in the fingers, while gnawing was used for movement pain in the shoulders. The findings of this study raise an interesting question about whether arthritis patients are registering pain on movement or at rest when they complete the MPQ. Standard instructions for the use of the MPQ need to be agreed to ensure that the results of future studies of RA pain are comparable in the light of these findings. In a subsequent paper Badley and Papageorgiou (1989) reported that they found no evidence to support the idea that the overall assessment of RA pain is dominated by the pain of the most painful joint, or that some joints contribute more to overall pain than others. Very little seems to be known about the cognitive synthesis of multiple joint pains in the process of making such overall judgements.

Far less is known about the language of stiffness. Rhind *et al.* (1980) interviewed a hundred patients about their stiffness and found spontaneous descriptions of sensations in the joints which included movement difficulties, pain, functional difficulties, abnormal sensations and stiffness. The majority indicated limitations to their range of movement when asked to say which word best described their stiffness. Helliwell *et al.* (1993) offered a menu of eight definitions to fifty-nine RA patients, but also those with OA and healthy people. They found that individuals with RA predominantly used the expressions resistance to movement (31 per cent), limited range (31 per cent) and lack of movement (20 per cent) to define their stiffness. The fifty healthy people who were all health professionals also preferred these three expressions and in particular resistance to movement, indicating that patient and professional appear to speak a similar language where stiffness is concerned. Who learns it from whom is not apparent, but it raises interesting social issues about how language is shared and shaped in medical contexts.

Some measures of arthritis pain have been developed within quality of life scales as part of a more global assessment of the impact of disease (see Chapter 4 for a thorough description of QoL measures). The Arthritis Impact Measurement Scales (AIMS) (Meenan *et al.*, 1980) included symptom assessment within the nine subscales of the original fifty-five items. Pain is evaluated by four reliable items in the long version and two items in a short form (Wallston, *et al.,* 1989).

In the development of the original AIMS, pain was correlated with patients' perceptions of health and of their disease activity. But pain level was poorly correlated with the doctor's three reports of functional activity, disease activity and joint count, revealing striking differences between doctors' and patients' perceptions of the condition. Meenan *et al.* suggest that doctors and patients focus on different aspects of health status when trying to summarise the condition. However, this discrepancy does raise a fundamental conceptual issue about whether doctors can truly 'know' what their patients are experiencing, even with communications at their very best. This research unambiguously demonstrates that the most valuable mode of assessment in the end is to ask the patient.

Further investigations of the properties of the AIMS have confirmed that the pain items are highly loaded as an important factor within the scale. It is therefore a distinctive identifiable component of the condition in the AIMS, rather than being subsumed as in the Sickness Impact Profile (Chapter 5). Pain is well correlated with some physical conditions which are considered to be an index of severity, such as joint count. Over a 6 month period, changes in patients' overall perceptions and changes in pain score were highly correlated and showed good test–retest reliability (Meenan *et al.*, 1982).

Recent publication of the revised AIMS2 shows that the scales have been reorganised to form twelve scales of seventy-eight items. Items in the original nine scales have been reduced to a maximum of five, scaling problems have been resolved and new scales of work, social support and arm function have been included. Perhaps more innovative is the inclusion of three new areas of assessment which look at the impact of arthritis on each area of health, satisfaction with each area and a prioritisation page where participants can identify three areas where they would most like to see health improvements (Meenan *et al.*, 1992). This new emphasis on the subjective assessment of goals and priorities provides a much more comprehensive assessment than has hitherto been available. These quality of life measures enable pain and discomforts to be assessed within the context of the many other psychosocial and physical aspects of the disease.

The search for an 'objective' method of measurement may have been an impediment to the progress of cognitive behaviour therapy. The use of subjective reports does not have the ethical problems inherent in the observational method of obtaining data without the patient's consent. Research based on Keefe and Block's much-cited categorisation of pain behaviours provides an example of how this method has been used in evaluating the success of cognitive behaviour therapy; a prime goal of neo-behaviourist treatment is the reduction of these pain behaviours. McDaniel *et al.* (1986), carried out four experiments to assess the reliability of observing patients performing standard manoeuvres like sitting, standing, walking and reclining. Trained observers recorded grimacing, active and passive rubbing, holding the body rigid with excessive stiffness, guarding movements, self-stimulation through repetitive movements and so on. However no measures of cognitions were taken to find out why participants believed they had carried out these movements, so leaving such actions open to speculation and potential misinterpretation. More recently this method has not been relied on as the sole outcome measure, but is used along with other measures of self-report which in some cases appear to reflect similar outcome trends (e.g. Bradley *et al.*, 1985). This is not to say that 'objective' measures should be discarded, just that in the treatment of chronic pain 'what people say is just as important as what they do, even though the two do not always correspond' (Linton, 1985: 293).

When patients are aware that they are being observed they change their behaviour in many subtle ways. Anderson *et al.* (1992) found that patients who knew they were being videoed during a physical examination behaved differently to those who were unaware. However, social facilitation is predicated on the assumption that behaviour changes when others are present; an audience effect is to be expected. What does not seem to have been tested is whether the behaviour of chronic pain patients with RA changes any more or less than that of pain-free people in similar circumstances, namely when others – in this case health professionals – are visibly making judgements. Furthermore it is difficult to know how far assessments obtained in these studies were contaminated by patients' suspicions. More important from a clinical viewpoint is that if decisions about care are made on the basis of private information collected unknowingly, how does this affect the desired trusting therapeutic relationship between patient and health professional?

SUMMARY

Pain and stiffness are two important clinical features of rheumatoid arthritis. Pain is a powerful motivator (Melzack and Dennis, 1978) and is a central reason why people seek help for their condition and comply with aggressive treatments and their side-effects. New research on inflammation and the plasticity of neurons has direct implications for the understanding and treatment of pain in this disease. While it is important to continue investigating the biological mechanisms responsible for generating discomfort in this condition, there is a growing body of data and theory to indicate that psychological processes and related sociodemographic factors may not have been attributed with the importance they deserve. New and improved methods of assessment are likely to act as a stimulus to increased research in this area.

Chapter 5

Quality of life

As discussed in the previous chapter it is increasingly recognised that chronic illnesses such as rheumatoid arthritis may have such pervasive effects upon the individual's life that, in addition to considering conventional clinical and laboratory measures of disease progression, it is equally important to assess these broader impacts. There are a number of distinct but overlapping terms intended to convey such broader consequences of disease; 'functional status', 'health status' and 'subjective health status' are commonly used alternatives to refer to personal experiences arising from disease. One might also refer to the concepts of impairment, disability and handicap developed by the WHO (1980) to refer to the distinct levels of broader disadvantage beyond bodily disease processes. Alongside such concepts there has emerged a growing body of evidence regarding chronic illness that uses the framework of 'quality of life' to take account of consequences of disease for daily life (Hopkins, 1992; Walker and Rosser, 1993). The assessment of quality of life in RA is the subject of this chapter.

DIMENSIONS OF QUALITY OF LIFE

Despite the enormous expansion of research on quality of life in the field of health care in the last 20 years, the concept has never been clearly defined and, like other social scientific constructs, it is somewhat broad and open-ended in range of referents. One review concluded that aspects of quality of life in medical studies could be classified into one of thirteen dimensions: emotional well-being, spirituality, sexuality, social functioning, family life, occupational functioning, communication, eating, functional ability, physical status, treatment satisfaction, future orientation and global ratings of life satisfaction (Cella and Tulsky, 1990). In practice, the majority of studies of chronic disease concentrate on a much narrower range of aspects of quality of life: physical function and symptoms, social well-being and psychological well-being (Fitzpatrick, Fletcher, *et al.*, 1992). These categories will be used here although, as will become clear throughout the book, in reality such divisions impose somewhat arbitrary boundaries in relation to the realities of chronic illness. This chapter considers the range of impacts RA may have on individuals and the ways in which quality of life measures attempt to assess such impacts.

Physical function, pain and fatigue

Estimates of the impact of RA on individuals' lives vary according to characteristics of patient groups studied and measures used to assess quality of life or related concepts. If we look more broadly at musculoskeletal disorders, arthritis is the commonest cause of disability (Martin, Meltzer and Elliott, 1988). American, Canadian and British surveys produce a range of estimates from 5 per cent to 7 per cent of individuals in the general population experiencing substantial disability arising from musculoskeletal disorders (Badley, 1992). Amongst individuals in the community reporting self-defined arthritis, between 30 per cent and 60 per cent report some limitation arising from arthritis, depending on the precise measures of limitations used in the survey (Holbrook *et al.*, 1990; Verbrugge *et al.*, 1991). These limitations are most likely to involve problems of mobility around the house, ability to walk distances outside or use public transport. A small minority of people with RA are wheelchair or bed-bound. For the rest, walking may be both difficult and tiring. Individuals with RA also report being constantly concerned about falling when they do move around, so that they may further restrict their mobility.

Range of movement is also affected as pain, stiffness and lack of strength make the movement of the body from one position to another (for example in a chair or bed) very difficult. Movement is particularly difficult in the morning when stiffness is worst so that getting out of bed can be one of the most difficult tasks. A wide range of other functional difficulties may be experienced. In one study of patients with RA, 79 per cent experienced at least some degree of difficulty with housework tasks such as vacuuming, 68 per cent had difficulties in aspects of dressing such as tying shoelaces or doing up buttons; and 64 per cent had difficulties climbing a short flight of stairs or having a bath (Pincus *et al.*, 1983). Even tasks that are mundane and taken for granted by healthy individuals require special effort, planning and often dependence upon others, when performed by individuals with RA (see Chapter 3). The conservation of energy in order to handle everyday tasks is a common theme in patients' accounts of how they deal with disabilities (Bury, 1988).

Pain is a major consequence of RA and a primary concern for most patients. It is of central importance to an understanding of the disorder and is therefore considered in particular detail in the next chapter. It needs to be emphasised how central it is in discussions of the quality of life of patients with RA. Pain relief is the primary objective for patients with RA who seek medical help and is ranked by them as the most important symptom (Gibson and Clark, 1985). In comparative studies of different chronic illnesses, pain is the dimension of quality of life in terms of which patients with RA are most distinguishable from individuals with other major chronic health problems (Stewart *et al.*, 1989). It is common to find that severity of pain is the variable with the strongest relationship to psychological well-being among patients with RA (Hawley and Wolfe, 1988; Frank *et al.*, 1988). Severity of experienced pain is not well predicted by conventional disease variables in RA and there is a wide range of (potentially modifiable) psychosocial factors that are associated with the experience of pain.

Another symptom not so widely recognised but important for the quality of daily life of individuals with RA is fatigue. As has already been pointed out, the extra effort involved in carrying out basic tasks involving mobility or movement tires individuals with RA to a greater extent than their healthy counterparts. Fatigue is a primary symptom of RA and may be particularly debilitating when the disease is active. When one particular quality of life instrument, the Nottingham Health Profile, was administered to patients with RA, the most severe score of the six dimensions measured by the instrument was fatigue (Fitzpatrick, Ziebland, *et al.*, 1992). Fatigue is greater during flare-ups, during periods of emotional distress, or unusual levels of activity, and requires substantial adjustment on the part of the individual to preserve energy (Tack, 1990). Recent in-depth, qualitative research also suggests that patients with RA are able to recognise and describe a number of different 'types' of fatigue which require different coping strategies (Papageorgiou, 1994).

It is possible to see the extent and range of problems associated with RA by means of one of the quality of life instruments used widely in this and other areas of medicine. A number of surveys of individuals with RA have been carried out using an instrument called the Sickness Impact Profile (SIP: Bergner *et al.*, 1981) (Table 5.1).

Table 5.1 Dimensions of quality of life in various samples of patients with RA as indicated by Sickness Impact Profile

Dimension	*Individuals with RA*			*Comparison groups of well individuals*	
	Seattle, USA	London, UK	Gothenburg, Sweden	Seattle, USA	Gothenburg, Sweden
Walking	21.0	23.6	26.0	3.1	4.7
Body care & movement	12.7	21.1	19.3	1.0	2.8
Mobility	10.4	15.1	21.1	2.7	2.5
Work	46.5	35.2	41.7	8.5	2.6
Sleeping & rest	17.6	23.5	26.7	7.2	10.3
Eating	3.5	1.3	5.0	1.6	1.6
Housework	26.3	40.2	41.9	5.4	4.1
Recreation	26.7	26.7	31.2	10.2	13.8
Emotions	13.2	17.7	16.7	3.8	7.9
Social interaction	11.7	12.1	12.2	5.2	6.1
Alertness	13.0	7.4	7.6	4.0	5.0
Communication	6.9	5.9	7.4	1.1	1.4

Note: Higher scores indicate poorer quality of life.
Sources: Seattle (Deyo *et al.*, 1982); London (Fitzpatrick *et al.*, 1989); Gothenburg (Sullivan *et al.*, 1990).

These studies have involved samples of patients in whom definite rheumatoid arthritis has been diagnosed. It is clear from these studies that patients with RA in a number of different countries differ from healthy comparison groups across a number of different dimensions of quality of life. For example, data from studies using the SIP confirm that patients with RA experience particular problems with regard to walking. Closer consideration of individual questionnaire items from the SIP show that a majority of patients with RA will affirm that they 'walk more slowly' and 'walk shorter distances or stop to rest often' (Deyo *et al.*, 1982).

The advantage of standard instruments such as the SIP is that they begin to address a much wider range of problems of quality of life that may arise from major health conditions. From studies such as those summarised in Table 5.1 one begins to obtain, as the instrument's title implies, a profile of the widest range of problems associated with particular diseases. For example, it is clear that housework is also a source of problems in all samples, with a majority of respondents affirming specific items such as 'not doing heavy work around the house' and 'doing less of regular daily work around the house'. The SIP also draws attention to the extent to which samples of respondents experience problems with their leisure activities. A majority affirm that they go out for entertainment less often because of their RA. Problems with sleep and rest are also common with nearly half affirming a specific statement that they sleep less at night.

Social well-being

Instruments such as the SIP also spell out the extent of problems associated with employment. Particularly severe consequences may arise in relation to employment after the onset of RA. Over one half of individuals with RA who worked before the onset of the disease stop work within 10 years of diagnosis (Yelin *et al.*, 1980). The income of individuals with RA is therefore considerably reduced. According to one study in the USA, men with RA had 48 per cent and women 27 per cent of the income of those without the disease (Mitchell *et al.*, 1988). The nature of the job held by the individual appears to be a better predictor of whether the individual becomes unemployed following disease onset than are biomedical variables such as disease severity. Those individuals holding jobs with work autonomy and flexibility are more likely to remain in employment after onset of RA (Yelin *et al.*, 1980). Individuals in professional or managerial occupations are considerably more likely to stay in employment after onset of RA (Callahan *et al.*, 1992). Conventional rheumatological measures of disease made no additional contribution to explaining job loss in this sample.

For those who manage to continue in paid employment the difficulties may be substantial. Individuals with RA may have to rely on others at work for help at work tasks, with the consequent feelings of dependency, or alternatively may seek to conceal pain or difficulties arising from work tasks (Locker, 1983). Tasks may require extra time to be carried out and flare-ups may result in problems of time-keeping at work. However, the accounts provided by those who were unemployed because of RA make clear the various losses arising from job loss (Locker, 1983). As well as the immediate financial problems arising from reduced income, individuals experienced a diminished sense of autonomy, and a loss of the various personal incentives to 'carry on' that work had provided. There is other evidence to suggest that an absence of paid employment for individuals with RA is deleterious. In a study of 723 patients attending clinics for RA, those without paid employment reported higher levels of pain and depression, even when confounding factors such as disease severity were controlled for (Fifield *et al.*, 1991).

Domestic roles

Women still carry out a disproportionate share of domestic work and many view their role in the home as an important part of their identity. As RA is more common amongst women, it is important to examine the impact that the disease may have on domestic roles. Reisine and her colleagues distinguish between two different aspects of womens' domestic lives that may be affected by RA: their instrumental and nurturing functions (Reisine *et al.*, 1987). The majority of women with RA in their study experienced limitations in their instrumental roles; for example, 73 per cent had some limitations in cleaning the house, 65 per cent in laundry work and 61 per cent in shopping. By nurturing roles, Reisine and colleagues refer to the roles, predominantly taken on by women, of giving attention and support to other household members and maintaining family ties with others outside the household such as relatives and friends. Although not as extensively affected as instrumental roles, nevertheless 42 per cent reported that RA had limited their ability to maintain family ties with others and 39 per cent were limited in their ability to look after friends or family when they were sick. Overall satisfaction with their lives was more affected by limitations in their nurturing roles than in instrumental activities. Along with the distress associated with being unable to fulfil nurturing roles in the household is the sense of having to be helped or cared for by others and the problems of dependency and non-reciprocity in family relationships that RA can impose (Locker, 1983; see Chapter 3 for an account of this).

Family and social life

The results of the studies using the SIP in Table 5.1 also indicate potential problems in relation to social relationships. More detailed discussion of the significance of social relations in RA is provided in another chapter (see Chapter 8). However there is an interesting and unresolved question as to whether and to what extent patients with RA do experience problems in their various social relations as a consequence of the illness.

First let us consider close relations such as marriage. Some studies, relying largely on the evidence from demographic variables alone, have investigated whether rates of divorce are elevated amongst individuals with RA. These studies, however, have proved inconclusive and even where apparently higher rates of divorce have been found among individuals with RA, the majority of divorces *preceded* the onset of disease (Anderson *et al.*, 1985). More detailed descriptive studies of the lives of individuals with RA emphasise the various frictions and frustrations that occur in marriages involving a partner with RA, arising from dependency, shared problems of isolation or reduced income (Locker, 1983; Williams, 1987). The most frequent source of family problems in Locker's study was the pain experienced by individuals with RA. RA patients stated that their pain made them irritable and bad-tempered in ways that constantly threatened to affect family relationships. Reisine and colleagues (1987) found that interest and activity in sex was adversely affected for 53 per cent of women in their sample.

Studies that have attempted to examine the consequences of RA for family life using more quantitative measures and comparison groups have found rather different evidence. Earle and colleagues (1979) compared patients with RA to a comparison group of well individuals on a standardised measure of the respondent's feelings of 'family appreciation' and found no differences. Similarly a study of 158 patients with RA using a well-established measure of social relationships, the Interview Schedule for Social Interaction (Henderson *et al.*, 1980), found that individuals with RA rated their close attachment relationships, the majority of which were with family, at least as favourably as other well comparison groups (Fitzpatrick *et al.*, 1988). Moreover, this positive view of the quality of close attachment relationships was not reduced among respondents who had more severe disease either in terms of self-report or rheumatological measures.

It is clear that the impact of RA on family life may be more dynamic and varied than can be conveyed by such measures. One study suggested that whilst individuals with RA did not differ from other comparison groups in terms of feeling supported by their families, they felt less able to participate in or enjoy family activities (Rudick *et al.*, 1992). In the study by Earle and colleagues (1979), older individuals with RA were more likely to feel appreciated by the family. As Locker points out (1983), when onset of RA is later in life, marital and family relationships are stabilised so that the many demands posed by the disease are less disruptive to these strong relationships. However, for widowed women with RA, the illness has even greater costs in terms of reduced sources of support and increased levels of distress and depression (Fitzpatrick *et al.*, 1991).

Individuals' relations with friends are more clearly at risk with onset of RA. Over half of a sample of individuals with RA reported that they go out less often to visit people because of their disease (Deyo *et al.*, 1982). On standardised instruments, individuals with RA report fewer opportunities for contact with friends and acquaintances and less satisfaction with these relationships (Fitzpatrick *et al.*, 1988). As the disease becomes more severe, such contacts and friendships become further eroded. Reduced mobility makes social relations outside the home more difficult to maintain. The very effort involved to get out is a strong disincentive. In some cases social withdrawal may arise because the individual prefers to avoid stigma and embarrassment associated with her condition (Locker, 1989; Williams and Wood, 1987). For whatever reasons, changes in social relationships that may follow onset of RA pose a major threat to the individual's well-being and quality of life (Fitzpatrick *et al.*, 1991; Patrick *et al.*, 1986).

Psychological well-being

An important dimension of quality of life in RA is psychological well-being. The major focus of research on psychological well-being has been on depression. Within this research it has been customary for an absence of depression to be associated with positive psychological well-being. It is both convenient and somewhat naive to assume that the absence of depression or the absence of high levels of depressed mood can be equated with psychological well-being (Wallston and DeVellis 1991). This approach also begs the question as to what the exact nature of positive psychological well-being is. Some alternative approaches have been developed which involve measuring other psychological dimensions. These have included measures of self esteem such as the Rosenberg Scale (Rosenberg, 1965) and the General Positive Affect subscale of the Mental Health Inventory (Veit and Ware, 1983). The focus of this section will be on depression and its assessment in RA as this is where the bulk of research has been performed.

Methodological issues

Besides the conceptual issues as to how psychological well-being is defined, as discussed above, there are a number of other methodological issues that need to be considered. One of the most important is the manner of assessment. Essentially two categories of technique exist for the assessment for depression.

Self-administered questionnaires are frequently used to assess depression. There are a number of instruments, including the Beck Depression Inventory, the Zung depression Scale, the Hospital Anxiety and Depression Scale, The General Health Questionnaire, CSD 90 and the Middlesex Hospital Questionnaire. The measurement of depressive symptoms by means of self-report questionnaires is not considered adequate for diagnosing clinical depression (Rodin, 1991). Although cut-off points have been agreed on many scales these have not been standardised on the appropriate medical samples in most cases (DeVellis, 1993). Besides these scales, which are widely used in a range of conditions, some researchers have used the depression scales from commonly used arthritis measures such as the AIMS (Hawley and Wolfe, 1993). Some comparisons have been performed between arthritis-based measures such as the AIMS and depression indices.

For example Blalock *et al.* report a correlation of 0.81 between the CES-D and the depression subscale of the AIMS (Blalock *et al.*, 1989). Attempts to define cut-off points on the AIMS is a considerably more difficult task (see Hawley and Wolfe, 1993).

The validity of these instruments for use in RA has also been brought into question in that many have 'disease-related' items such as fatigue and sleep disturbance, which are appropriate for use in psychiatric populations, but are problematic for use with physically ill individuals (Bradley 1989a). These items reflect the degree of physical illness and lead to an inflated score on the depression inventory (Peck *et al.*, 1989, Pincus *et al.*, 1986). Blalock *et al.*, however, found that although certain items in the CES-D did appear to reflect the disease process, the degree of overestimation of depression if these were included was modest. (Blalock *et al.*, 1989).

An alternative to questionnaire assessment is the use of standardised psychiatric assessments which may be used to compare the incidence of depression as assessed by structured interview. Common amongst these is the Clinical Interview Schedule, the Diagnostic Interview Schedule and the Psychiatric Assessment Schedule. Creed, in his review of the area, claims that it is only with a formal interview by someone trained on the instrument that an accurate measure of the evidence of depression may be obtained (Creed, 1990). Studies have indicated that formal interview techniques do produce a lower incidence of patients with depression (see Table 5.2).

Table 5.2 Prevalence studies of depression in RA

Author	*n*	*Instrument*	*% Prevalence*	*Comments*
Zaphiropoulos & Burry (1974)	50	BDI	46 (admission) 23 (discharge)	Inpatients
Gardiner (1980)	129	GHQ	53.5 (discharge)	Inpatients
Bishop *et al.* (1987)	39	BDI	19 (admission)	Inpatients
Chandarana *et al.* (1987)	86	GHQ HAD	32 28	Outpatients
Murphy *et al.* (1988)	80	PAS	21	In and outpatients
Frank *et al.* (1988)	137	DIS	17	Outpatients
Blalock *et al.* (1989)		CESD AIMS	30–46	Outpatients
Hawley & Wolfe (1992)	1152	AIMS	20–37	Outpatients

In order to examine whether individuals with RA have a raised incidence of depression, comparisons have been made to incidence rates in the general population. In general these studies have indicated a higher incidence of depression in individuals with RA (DeVellis, 1993).

Comparisons to individuals with other clinical conditions have found similar rates of depression (Frank *et al.*, 1988; Murphy *et al.*, 1988; DeVellis, 1993). Thus while individuals with RA have higher rates of depression than the general population they do not differ from other clinical samples. Some clinicians have suggested that, because RA is a long-term condition which involves much joint destruction and associated pain and disability, of all the rheumatological conditions it is most likely to lead to depression. Hawley and Wolfe (1992) compared the incidence of depression and depressed mood in a large group of individuals with a variety of rheumatic conditions and found no evidence to support the notion that RA patients, in comparison to individuals with other rheumatological conditions, have a particular propensity to develop depression.

Although individuals with RA do not appear to have higher rates of depression or levels of depressed mood in comparison to individuals with other clinical conditions it remains important to establish what factors influence psychological well-being. The most simple prediction is that the physical manifestations of the disease lead to the development of depression. Studies have, however, failed to find a direct relationship between the physical markers of the disease and clinical depression or depressed mood (Creed 1990; Newman *et al.*, 1989; Blalock and DeVellis, 1992). Evidence has been accumulating that the impact of RA is mediated through a number of psychological and social factors. Notable amongst these are coping responses and social supports. The mediating role of these factors is discussed in later chapters in this volume (see Chapters 7 and 8).

It is important to recognise that the impact of RA on psychological well-being is a process that is likely to change over time. Some have postulated a general process across all chronic illnesses whereby psychological well-being improves over time (Cassileth *et al.*, 1984). In RA there is some evidence for this process of adaptation over time which may either be directly observed (Cassileth *et al.*, 1984) or is only apparent if the relationship between psychological well-being and disease-duration is examined after statistically controlling for deterioration over time in disease severity (Deyo, Inui, *et al.*, 1982; Newman *et al.*, 1989).

It is possible that available measures of psychological well-being used in studies of RA are limited and fail to recognise more common but less frank forms of distress. We are beginning to assess the extent of forms of distress other than depression and anxiety, such as feelings of helplessness, uncertainty, loss of control, reduced self-esteem and impaired body image that may occur in RA (Burckhardt, 1985; Fitzpatrick *et al.*, 1990). Such forms of distress are not explicable by or reducible to more conventional psychiatric categories, but are a substantial potential contribution to reduced quality of life.

Another important factor needs to be considered in the context of quality of life. Depressed mood is generally associated with very dramatically reduced perceptions of quality of life (Sensky and Catalan, 1992). In a major population-based survey, individuals with clearly established depression were found to have scores for physical, emotional and role functioning that were as bad as or sometimes worse than those found in eight major chronic medical illnesses (Wells *et al.*, 1989). The study concluded that depression should be considered as a major disabling disorder. It is unclear whether depression directly affects functioning or rather *perceptions* of function (Brooks *et al.*, 1990). There are studies that show similar effects of psychological mood on general functioning in RA (Spiegel *et al.*, 1988). It is clear from such evidence that patients with RA and poor psychological mood may be a particularly problematic group both in terms of assessment and care.

THE ASSESSMENT OF QUALITY OF LIFE

Few fields of medicine have witnessed as much effort to assess the quality of life of patients as has rheumatology. The degree of emphasis on self-reported experiences of patients partly reflects the fact that none of the conventional rheumatological measures of disease process and outcome clearly commands consensus. In addition the efficacy of drug therapy and other treatments is so modest that the search for sensitive and appropriate outcome measures has been particularly pressing. Above all the patient's and doctor's perceptions of global aspects of disease impact are relied upon in clinical practice to assess progress. Therefore systematic measures of such perceptions are essential. Increasingly it has been recognised that patients can provide accurate and informative reports of the diverse range of experiences of their disease and its impact on their lives and that these can be used alongside conventional medical measures to assess progress. We first consider the development and range of such measures before finally examining their various potential or actual contributions.

Initially, assessments of the patient's general condition in rheumatology were quite narrow. The earliest and still widely used measure of a patient's general status in rheumatology is what are known as the Steinbrocker criteria for classifying level of functional impairment adopted by the American College of Rheumatology (Steinbrocker *et al.*, 1949). This involves classification of patients into one of four broad categories as listed in Table 5.3.

Table 5.3 The Steinbrocker criteria for classification of functional impairment

Class I	Complete functional capacity with ability to carry on all usual duties without handicaps
Class II	Functional capacity adequate to conduct normal activities despite handicap of discomfort or limited mobility of one or more joints
Class III	Functional capacity adequate to perform only little or none of the duties of usual occupation or self-care
Class IV	Largely or wholly incapacitated, with patient bedridden or confined to wheelchair, permitting little or no self-care

Source: Steinbrocker *et al.*, 1949.

This simple classification system resembles other early attempts to assess patients with other diseases in global terms, for example the Karnofsky Performance Index used in oncology and rehabilitation (Karnofsky and Burchenal, 1949), or the New York Heart Association's four-point functional classification (Harvey *et al.*, 1974). Such scales are limited for various reasons. They may contain too few scale points so that there is little scope to discriminate between patients or detect change over time. They are unidimensional, whereas it is clear that dimensions of quality of life can be independent. They do not include psychosocial aspects of well-being. Above all they are for clinicians to complete. In view of the considerable evidence of discrepancies in judgements between health professionals and their patients, most methods of assessing quality of life now depend on the patient's report (Sprangers and Aaronson, 1992).

Patient-based measures

All of the measures considered in the rest of this chapter are based on patients' responses. Most can be administered by interview, but increasingly, for reasons of economy, they are intended for self-completion. Three main types of instrument will be considered: disease-specific, generic and individualised measures. Disease-specific instruments have been developed to be used in a narrow range of diseases, in the current case, arthritis. Generic instruments, by contrast, are intended to be used in the widest range of health problems. Individualised instruments may in principle work in both applications.

Disease-specific measures

The Health Assessment Questionnaire

The first major instrument developed to measure the patient's experience of RA was the Health Assessment Questionnaire (HAQ) (Fries *et al.*, 1982). It was originally conceived as an 'outcome' measure to contrast with existing measures in rheumatology such as ESR and joint counts, which were considered by Fries and colleagues as 'process measures' (Fries *et al.*, 1982). The core instrument contains two elements, a disability index and a pain scale. The disability index consists of twenty items to assess the following eight functions: dressing and grooming, arising, eating, walking, hygiene, reach, grip and outside activity. Individuals assess their degree of difficulty (on a scale from 'no difficulty' to 'unable to do') with each of the items. Scores from each of the eight components are averaged to create a disability index with a range from 0 to 3. Pain is measured with a visual analogue scale. This instrument is the simplest and shortest of commonly used measures and is probably the most widely used. A more recent version of the HAQ, the 'modified HAQ' was developed because it was felt that two of the four responses in the HAQ, 'with some difficulty' and 'with much difficulty', might actually disguise a wide range of levels of disability and also because patients might use these same response categories over time despite experiencing substantial change (Pincus *et al.*, 1983). The modified HAQ therefore asks patients about a shorter number of items (8) but, in addition, includes questions about satisfaction and change with regard to each function. A recent study has provided evidence that the change questions in the modified HAQ do indeed provide more precise and sensitive measures of degrees of change experienced by the patient that are not registered in the conventional format (Ziebland *et al.*, 1992).

The Arthritis Impact Measurement Scales

The Arthritis Impact Measurement Scales (AIMS) were also conceived as outcome measures to complement measures of disease activity (Meenan, 1982). It was felt that existing functions and activities of daily living scores did not take account of the full range of aspects of the WHO's model of health as a physical, psychological and social state. The instrument that emerged consists of forty-five items over nine dimensions of mobility, physical activity, activities of daily living, dexterity, household activities, pain, depression, anxiety and social activities. Items vary in terms of response format; some involve 'yes' or 'no' choices, whereas other items require selecting the degree of help required for a task (from 'without help' to 'completely unable to . . .') or the frequency with which something is experienced ('always' to 'never'). Nevertheless, scoring is simple with items within a scale summed and then normalised to a 0–10 range. An item about sexual activity was originally included but dropped because of low response rates (Meenan *et al.*, 1982). Five underlying dimensions were revealed through factor analysis: lower extremity function, upper extremity function, mood, symptoms (mainly pain) and social interaction (Mason *et al.*, 1988). Like the HAQ the AIMS has undergone modifications and a more recent version (AIMS2) has added three dimensions; arm function, work and social support (Meenan *et al.*, 1992).

Several other disease-specific instruments have been developed. The Toronto Questionnaire is a fifty-six-item questionnaire which focuses on physical function and activities of daily living (Helewa *et al.*, 1982). The McMaster Health Index Questionnaire (Chambers *et al.*, 1982), is a sixty-nine-item questionnaire which assesses physical, emotional and social function. Unlike the HAQ and AIMS, which were developed by American groups, as their names imply the Toronto and McMaster instruments were developed by Canadian groups and have received far less general research attention.

Generic measures

The Sickness Impact Profile

The most established and widely used generic instrument is the Sickness Impact Profile (SIP) (Bergner *et al.*, 1981). The SIP consists of 136 simple statements (for example 'I only stand for short periods of time') with 'yes' or 'no' responses. Items are summed into one of twelve dimensions as indicated in Table 5.1. Scores in the dimensions of walking, body care and movement and mobility may be further summed to form a physical scale and the dimensions of emotions, social interaction, alertness and communication may be summed to form a psychosocial scale. The SIP has been used quite extensively in relation to RA (Deyo *et al.*, 1982; Ahlmen *et al.*, 1988; Fitzpatrick *et al.*, 1989). One of the main problems with generic instruments such as the SIP is that they may contain items of no great relevance to the particular disorder under study. It has been suggested that the eating and communication dimensions can be dropped in the context of RA with little loss of relevant information (Deyo *et al.*, 1983; Sullivan *et al.*, 1990).

Quality of Well-being scale

The Quality of Well-being (QWB) scale is another generic instrument designed to measure quality of life. It was originally intended to be used either in interview format or for self-completion but is now only recommended for use with an interviewer as it requires filter questions and the necessity for an interviewer to probe to obtain precise responses (Kaplan *et al.*, 1993). The instrument consists of two sections. The first section assesses functional states in relation to three dimensions: mobility, physical activity and social activity. The mobility and physical activity scales distinguish among three levels of function and the social activity scale among five levels. The second section assesses specific symptom or problem complexes (e.g. various symptoms such as stiffness or pain, are present). These states and symptoms have preference weights that reflect the values of a general population in San Diego, California. These weights reflect both the severity of disease and disability as well as their temporal impact on quality of life. The weighted scores are added from the two sections and provide an overall score for any individual with a range from 0 to 1. The instrument's weights have been recalculated using a sample of RA patients to be more relevant to this population (Balaban *et al.*, 1986). The instrument has been used in a major clinical trial in RA (Bombardier *et al.*, 1986). It is questionable whether the QWB scale will prove informative in relation to conditions such as RA because the assessment of functional states permits distinctions between only a small number of very broad levels of function.

Other generic scales

There are a number of other generic instruments that have been applied to RA. In particular the SF-36 is a thirty-six-item questionnaire with scales assessing physical functioning, role limitations due to physical problems, social functioning, bodily pain, general mental health, role limitations due to emotional problems, vitality and general health perceptions (Ware and Sherbourne, 1992). An early form of the instrument was used to describe a range of chronic health problems including arthritis (Stewart *et al.*, 1989). A similar short form of instrument is the Nottingham Health Profile (NHP) which has thirty-eight items with 'yes' or 'no' responses, contributing to one of six scales: energy, pain, emotional reactions, sleep, social isolation and physical mobility (McEwen, 1993). It has been used in one study of rheumatoid arthritis (Fitzpatrick, Ziebland, *et al.*, 1992).

Several of the quality of life instruments discussed (the Sickness Impact Profile, the Quality of Well-being scale and the Nottingham Health Profile) use explicit weights to assess the severity or desirability of items included in the instruments. These weights are obtained from experimental panels' assessments. A study of patients with RA found that the SIP and NHP were no more sensitive if these weights were replaced by simpler values (Jenkinson *et al.*, 1991).

Individualised quality of life measures

A third kind of approach to the assessment of quality of life has begun to find favour in recent years, particularly in the field of arthritis. A number of groups have argued that standard quality of life instruments may be too insensitive to the subtle changes produced by arthritis therapies. They may contain many items that may not be relevant to any particular individual. They also do not allow for variation in the salience or significance of particular functions or aspects of daily life to different individuals.

The MACTAR Patient Preference Disability Questionnaire

In the MACTAR instrument individuals are asked to identify which activities are affected by their arthritis (Tugwell *et al.*, 1987). They then rank the different activities nominated. These then constitute a baseline state of disability for each individual against which to measure change over time. In some versions of MACTAR such change is scored quite simply for each nominated function (+1 for improvement, 0 for no change and –1 for deterioration) (Tugwell *et al.*, 1990). In other versions more continuous measurement of change over time is provided by having patients use a visual analogue scale to express change in individualised functions (Tugwell *et al.*, 1991). All of the patients studied have proved able to identify at least five areas of personal concern in relation to RA.

The Schedule for the Evaluation of Individual Quality of Life

This instrument (SEIQoL) was developed to assess individuals' personal priorities and goals in relation to quality of life (O'Boyle *et al.*, 1992). As with the MACTAR, individuals select five areas of life of personal importance in the context of a structured interview. To elicit the relative importance of the areas selected, respondents use a visual analogue scale to rate the QoL of hypothetical vignettes which involve the selected dimensions. Subjects also rate their own current status on the selected dimensions. Most importantly, although the instrument is intended for use in health research, and has been used with patients with severe osteoarthritis, individuals are not required to select health-related aspects of quality of life. Indeed patients with OA selected social, leisure and family areas before health concerns. In this sense of not being confined to health-related quality of life, this approach differs from all others discussed so far.

ASSESSING QUALITY OF LIFE MEASURES

Strong claims are made for the measures of quality of life that have been discussed in this chapter. It may be argued that there is an element of grandiose hyperbole in claiming that they assess such a broad and abstract phenomenon as 'quality of life'. Even in more modest terms, these measures purport to assess the personal impact of ill-health. Such claims to measurement need to be examined in the same way as any other social-scientific or medical measure.

Reliability and validity

The reliability of an instrument is generally considered easier to examine than its validity. Reliability is an expression of the extent to which it yields the same results under the same conditions (Cox *et al.*, 1992). Most of the instruments that have been cited in this chapter have been examined for reliability but potential users should always check for evidence for this and other psychometric properties before adopting a particular measure for use. Studies of the AIMS instrument illustrate tests for reliability (Meenan *et al.*, 1982). For example, a sample of 625 patients with arthritis from ten different states in the USA completed the AIMS twice with a two-week interval. The lowest test–retest correlation coefficient for the nine scales was 0.84, which is quite acceptable. The most common alternative method of examining reliability was also examined: internal consistency, which examines whether the items in a scale are assessing the same theoretical construct. Again the coefficients of internal agreement for the nine AIMS scales were all above 0.7 and considered favourable.

An instrument may be reliable but not valid. In fact it may reliably fail to measure what it purports to measure! Validity is particularly hard to measure with quality of life constructs as there can be no gold standard against which to assess any particular instrument. A number of different approaches are required to inspect this aspect of a measure. One very important but necessarily informal approach is to consider face or content validity. The content of instruments can be examined in terms of whether it appears to be appropriate.

In reality, quality of life measures in the field of RA differ on this validity dimension in some obvious respects. For example, none of the disease-specific measures contain items specifically on fatigue, despite evidence that it is one of the main symptoms of the disease. As important are some of the more subtle differences among instruments. For example, in a number of AIMS items, in order for a respondent to score as having any degree of difficulty the individual has to report that they resort to some degree of help from someone else for that activity, for example, getting dressed. Comparable items in the HAQ also ask about the degree of difficulty, but individuals receive negative scores if *any* degree of difficulty is experienced. It is clear that in subtle ways the two instruments do measure different concepts of disability for the identical activities, with individuals having to become dependent on others in the case of the AIMS to register as having a problem in their daily activities (Ziebland *et al.*, 1993).

The more commonly cited evidence for validity tends to be on the basis of *construct validity*. Here one is concerned with whether scores on a measure have relationships with other variables that are consistent with what is theoretically known. A very common approach with many instruments, particularly for items that assess physical function, is to examine the extent to which scores for an instrument agree with more familiar clinical, radiological or laboratory measures of severity of disease, an approach adopted for the development of the AIMS (Meenan *et al.*, 1982) and the SIP in relation to RA (Deyo *et al.*, 1983). Ideally one should look for evidence of both *convergent* and *divergent* validity. For example, quality of life items assessing disabilities arising from upper limb function should correlate more with rheumatological measures of upper limb function, for example grip strength, and less with those concerned with lower limb function, such as observed walking time. In some instances elements of instruments assessing physical function can be validated by comparing scores with direct observation of patients' performance of relevant tasks (Sullivan *et al.*, 1987).

By comparison, the difficulties of validating measures of social and emotional well-being in quality of life instruments are substantial. Again convergent and divergent validity are critical. Measures of sociability should correlate more with other measures of the same construct and less with measures intended to assess psychological mood. The issue can be very important in the area of RA. For example, the ability to maintain social contacts has an important influence on individuals' well-being. The NHP has a scale – the social isolation scale – that measures this issue. However analysis of its relation to other variables suggests that the so-called social isolation scale may be more a measure of how individuals feel about themselves and their relations with others, a quite different construct (Fitzpatrick *et al.*, 1991).

Responsiveness

One of the most important requirements of quality of life instruments is that they be sensitive to any changes that occur in the individual's experience of her illness for better or worse. This property, referred to as 'responsiveness', has until recently received far less attention than issues of reliability and validity, despite the fact that, whether in drug trials or monitoring an individual patient's progress, it is important to distinguish real changes from measurement error.

There are a number of different methods of estimating an instrument's responsiveness and different methods can produce slightly different results (Deyo and Centor, 1986; Fitzpatrick *et al.*, 1993a). One approach is to examine the performance of an instrument in the context of a controlled drug trial to examine differences between an active drug and a placebo (Meenan *et al.*, 1984; Bombardier *et al.*, 1986). This method has been used to assess the responsiveness of a number of quality of life measures in RA. Of course this approach presupposes that the active drug should have such beneficial effects on quality of life. Usually other changes on other rheumatological measures of outcome in the active drug are required to support this assumption. A variant of this design is to examine quality of life measures in individuals who experience an intervention such as total hip replacement surgery, which is generally considered likely to improve a wide range of functions (Liang *et al.*, 1985). A second method is to examine the relationships between changes over time in quality of life and changes in other data available about patients. Typically this involves correlations between change scores for quality of life instruments being examined against changes in clinical or laboratory measures in disease activity (Meenan *et al.*, 1982; Sullivan *et al.*, 1990; Fitzpatrick *et al.*, 1993a). A final method is to examine changes over time in quality of life scores against the patient's own retrospective judgement that he or she has actually experienced a significant change over the time period covered. This method has been used in several studies of quality of life measures in RA (Deyo and Inui, 1984; Fitzpatrick *et al.*, 1989).

Comparative studies

A number of studies using one or more of the above methods have now been carried out comparing the responsiveness over time of two or more quality of life instruments in patients with arthritis. Overall, the similarities in these measures are more striking than the differences. Liang and colleagues (1985) compared five quality of life instruments (SIP, HAQ, AIMS, QWB, all discussed above together with the Functional Status Index (Jette, 1980)) in patients before and after total hip or knee replacement surgery. The criterion for evaluation was which instrument produced the greatest differences between administrations. Overall, no instrument produced consistently higher scores compared with the other instruments, although some differences in particular dimensions were noted. The HAQ and QWB did not appear to be particularly sensitive to improvements in mobility; the AIMS was insensitive to changes in social function that were identified by the other instruments. This lack of responsiveness of the AIMS social scale is commonly found (Meenan *et al.*, 1984; Anderson *et al.*, 1989; Fitzpatrick *et al.*, 1993a) and provides an important general observation. The social activity items primarily assess patterns of sociability such as frequency of contact with friends, and it is clear from a number of studies that such aspects of life are particularly slow to change in relation to other changes experienced by individuals with RA.

An observation found in several such studies is that generic instruments do not show markedly poorer responsiveness to change in RA compared to disease-specific instruments (Liang *et al.*, 1985; Fitzpatrick *et al.*, 1989; Weinberger *et al.*, 1992; Fitzpatrick *et al.*, 1993a). This is surprising, given that generic instruments are intended to be relevant to a wide range of health problems and therefore inevitably contain some items less relevant to people with RA. Some evidence suggests that the newer style individualised quality of life instruments may be more responsive to changes in RA compared to conventional disease-specific instruments (Tugwell *et al.*, 1991). However, a study of patients undergoing hip replacement surgery compared the SEIQoL individualised instrument with AIMS and found the latter more responsive to change over time (O'Boyle *et al.*, 1992).

Overall, there is still great scope for identifying means of improving responsiveness. There is evidence that patients with RA notice substantial changes over time (both improvements and deterioration) in their quality of life that are *not* detected by changes over time in existing quality of life instruments (Ziebland *et al.*, 1992). The evidence that patients do detect otherwise unmeasured changes in quality of life is provided by 'transition questions' in which patients directly assess change compared with a specific previous occasion (e.g. 'Compared with the last time you attended the clinic how would you rate your arthritis – better, the same or worse?'). Several studies have found that such direct questions may be very informative of changes for some aspects of quality of life (Mackenzie *et al.*, 1986; Tugwell *et al.*, 1990; Fitzpatrick *et al.*, 1993b).

USES OF QUALITY OF LIFE MEASURES

We have left until the end of the chapter the most important consideration of all, namely how the measures discussed here may be used. We consider three primary applications: basic understanding; outcome measures in clinical trials and evaluation; and clinical and practice applications.

Basic understanding

In many respects quality of life measures provide a missing link between disease processes and psychological and social processes. Most of the measures discussed in this chapter correlate with disease or psychological measures but rarely to such an extent that one is tempted to view them as redundant or explained away by disease or psychosocial processes. One of the most powerful applications of quality of life measures in RA has been to elucidate the long-term course of the disease in terms of personal impact. Wolfe and colleagues (1991) have examined clinic patients with RA over time using the HAQ, the depression and anxiety scales of AIMS, and various standard rheumatological measures. Disability as measured by the HAQ showed a constant rate of deterioration over a 22-year period, even though other measures such as ESR, stiffness and joint counts remained more stable. Interestingly, anxiety and depression in relation to RA did not show the same rate of deterioration as physical disability. This study provides further evidence of the progressive 'uncoupling' of disability and psychological well-being over time, suggested by other more cross-sectional data (Deyo *et al.*, 1982; Newman *et al.*, 1989). Equally important is the prognostic role that such instruments appear to play in a number of studies. Both the HAQ and the AIMS have been shown to be strongly predictive of the long-term course in terms of both disability and mortality in RA (Kazis *et al.*, 1990; Leigh and Fries, 1991, 1992; Wolfe and Cathey, 1991).

A second area in which these measures are beginning to permit important fundamental questions to be addressed is the relationship between disability and psychosocial processes. In many studies the relationship between disability and psychological variables is stronger than the relationship between disease and disability (McFarlane and Brooks, 1988; Newman *et al.*, 1989). Moreover, as is discussed in detail in a later chapter (Chapter 8), social support also appears to have an influence on whether individuals with RA deteriorate (Morgan, 1989). The direction of causal influences between psychological well-being, social support variables and disability is not yet clear and other chapters in this book will draw out some of the intriguing alternative possibilities. The important general point at this stage is the exciting potential for explanations provided by the measures discussed here.

Outcome measures in trials

Reference has already been made to the use of quality of life measures as outcomes in clinical trials. In the field of arthritis they have been used not only in the evaluation of drugs (Bombardier *et al.*, 1986; Tugwell *et al.*, 1990) but also surgery (Liang *et al.*, 1985) and alternative ways of providing care, for example in multidisciplinary teams (Ahlmen *et al.*, 1988) or home-based services (Helewa *et al.*, 1991). To date, the evidence of studies such as that of Wolfe and colleagues (1991) is not encouraging in terms of the beneficial effects of medical treatment on the course of disability and quality of life in arthritis, but the availability of more precise measures of outcome in the context of well-designed studies is still relatively new. The development of reliable patient-based measures of outcome is hailed by some as likely to transform the provision of health care.

Clinical and practice-based applications

Applications in clinical practice are still at an experimental stage compared with well-understood and informed usage in controlled trials. A number of practical applications have been identified. First, quality of life measures, because they are less expensive and labour intensive than clinical investigations, have been seen as a way of identifying more precisely the health needs of populations in order to improve planning and provision of services. It is undoubtedly the case that instruments like HAQ and AIMS would provide inexpensive and informative evidence of the prevalence of health problems in populations. Population-based surveys of health needs have begun to appear based on such instruments (Patrick and Peach, 1989). However, it is not clear whether the measures provide sufficiently precise data to fine-tune decisions about health care services (Frankel, 1991). Studies are needed to explore this application.

Some clinicians maintain that they use instruments such as HAQ routinely in their clinical care (Wolfe and Pincus, 1991). They argue that such applications are not expensive or disruptive and are invaluable in assisting clinical decisions. Unfortunately the one major trial to examine the benefits in terms of either clinical decisions or outcomes of patient satisfaction or health status, failed to detect any significant differences in either management or outcomes for patients with RA whose doctors received evidence of their patients' progress on quality of life measures compared to other patients where this did not occur (Kazis *et al.*, 1990). The authors suggest that information from quality of life scores was not fed back to doctors at the time when it might make a difference to clinical decisions. More positively, doctors found the information received from quality of life measures interesting. Perhaps the evidence of most relevance to future applications in a clinical context comes from a study in which patients expressed positive views about the benefits of their doctors receiving data about their progress from quality of life questionnaires (Nelson *et al.*, 1990). The majority of patients thought it was important for their doctor to have this information.

Although every individual's response to RA differs in important respects, and personal experiences subtly or dramatically fluctuate over time, some of this can be captured by the methods described in this chapter. With quality of life measures, vital information can be provided that complements other types of measurement.

Chapter 6

Patient–physician relationships

This chapter begins with a simple yet essential question: What does the patient want from a medical encounter with a physician? In the words of one physician:

> They [patients] want to be able to trust the competence and efficacy of their caregivers. They want to be able to negotiate the health care system effectively and to be treated with dignity and respect. Patients want to understand how their sickness or treatment will affect their lives, and they often fear that their doctors are not telling them everything they want to know. Patients worry about and want to learn how to care for themselves away from the clinical setting. They want us to focus on their pain, physical discomfort, and functional disabilities. They want to discuss the effect their illness will have on their family, friends, and finances. And they worry about the future.
>
> (Delbanco, 1992: 414)

The relationship between physicians and patients has been examined, probed and dissected since the early part of this century, although its roots go back much further. An early medical proverb warned *Dictim Premum Nocere* (First, do no harm). Before medicine was more science than art, physicians cultivated their bedside manner, as cures were often an impossibility and treatment had limited results. The elevation of science and technology to centre stage in the middle of this century downplayed the interpersonal aspects of health care, but there is a re-emerging interest in medicine as a social process. It is thus timely to bring back a comment made nearly 60 years ago, when a physician cautioned his colleagues that they could do as much harm to the patient with the slip of a word as with the slip of a knife

(Henderson, 1935). (Other than when a male physician is referred to, the pronouns of she and her will be used to refer to both patients and physicians in this chapter. Use of the masculine implies that most RA patients are male, which is not accurate, and that physicians should be.)

This chapter focuses on how the human-relations aspect of medicine affects adherence to prescribed treatment and satisfaction with medical care for patients with rheumatoid arthritis. These outcomes have been chosen primarily because they are assumed to affect health and quality of life (Kaplan *et al.*, 1989), and secondarily because the greatest amount of research has been done on these variables. The focus is on physicians because there has been little research on patients' relationships with health care professionals other than doctors, despite the fact that nurses, educators, physical therapists, occupational and recreational therapists, orthotists, psychologists and social workers play important if not critical roles in arthritis patient care. Whenever possible, research conducted with RA patients and their physicians, both rheumatologists and general practitioners, is presented, although in some areas it is necessary to draw on studies of other patient populations and practitioners. And, given that the majority of patients with RA are female and/or older, a section is devoted to how the patient's age and gender affect the patient–physician relationship.

THE PATIENT–PHYSICIAN RELATIONSHIP AS AN INTERPERSONAL TRANSACTION

In its most basic form, the patient–physician relationship is a dyadic interpersonal transaction. This conceptualisation was first presented by Bloom (1963) in what remains a classic text on the subject. Each participant brings to the medical encounter a different personal history, set of expectations, and conceptual framework. Each has a social and cultural context that shapes beliefs and actions. The roles of doctor and patient are patterns of expected behaviour, derived from both culture and individual experience. Thus, each player has some idea about how the other should act, but the patient–physician relationship is not often a symmetrical one (DiMatteo and DiNicola, 1982; DiMatteo and Hays, 1984). Physicians in Western society are socialised to dominate the doctor–patient interaction. For example, the physician sets the length and tone of the encounter; conversation is dominated by physicians using directed questions and declarative statements to control the flow and topic of conversation; physicians frequently ignore patients' questions or refer to patients by their first names (Conant, 1983). In these ways, physicians are able to command a good deal of authority, expertise and power over their patients. This power asymmetry may help patients follow prescribed treatment recommendations, of which the goal is better health, but it also provides a means of keeping people in their place (Waitzkin, 1983).

Adopting the idea that reality is socially constructed, Anderson and Helm (1979) portray the patient–physician encounter as 'a process of reality negotiation between frequently competing definitions of the situation' (pp. 261–2). That is, the patient–physician encounter involves a presentation of symptoms by the patient, followed by questioning, clarification of statements, a physical examination and clinical testing by the physician in order to arrive at a diagnosis (illness label), and treatment plan. In the process of reaching this end state, symptom descriptions are revised and the results of tests are integrated to clarify earlier accounts and lead to further explanation. Thus, the 'evidence' is socially constructed by both patient and physician. This process is necessary because of the great degree of uncertainty in medical diagnosis. As with any social situation, the participants are continually involved in impression management. Thus, the information presented by both participants may be erroneous, biased, or even irrelevant and the information received may be misunderstood, taken out of context, or even reinterpreted. Two case examples, one hypothetical and one real, will be used to illustrate this.

Case 1

A patient visits her physician complaining that she is in a good deal of pain despite the non-steroidal anti-inflammatory agents she has been taking faithfully. She is concerned that the treatment isn't working, but that it has created side-effects which are unpleasant and intrude on daily life. To her, it is a crisis, a problem that needs immediate attention. In contrast, this encounter is a routine one for the rheumatologist, who knows from current research and clinical experience that the drug may well cause such side-effects which can be remedied by anti-gastric medication. The physician nonchalantly explains to the patient that this happens frequently and writes out a new prescription for a reduced dosage of the medication, telling the patient that 'This should do it'. The patient accepts the prescription, but once home, takes only half the recommended dosage of medication because she believes it will continue to produce the side-effects. She also fails to keep her follow-up appointment.

As this case illustrates, different social constructions of the same symptoms or of the same treatment may lead to dissatisfaction and different decision-making on the part of patient or physician. The patient felt anxious about her future health and felt as if the physician was not listening to her concerns. After the visit, it was likely that she questioned the physician's expertise and was angry at the physician for not informing her of possible medication side-effects that would make her feel worse. She also felt that the physician was unconcerned about her psychological well-being. On the other hand, the physician felt that the patient was dramatising a mundane medical complaint and responded to her emotions defensively, by being uncommunicative and minimising the patient's concerns. In essence, the physician was responding to what she considered to be 'bad patient behaviour' (Lorber, 1979; Taylor, 1982). In this way, the emotions stemming from the different social constructions of the reality of the medical encounter may colour satisfaction with care, future interactions and adherence to the recommended treatment.

Case 2 (Conn, 1993)

A patient with moderate rheumatoid arthritis requiring disease-modifying drugs is given a choice of Plaquenil or injectable gold. The physician's preference is Plaquenil because it is less expensive and requires less monitoring, which suggests to the physician that it is more likely to be taken and therefore its efficacy will be more apparent. The patient, however, chooses gold injections, because a friend of hers is doing well with them.

In this case, the patient made a decision based on personal experience and not the physician's medical expertise. Despite his own preference, the physician acknowledged that the patient's high expectations of success with injectable gold were probably more salient for her in adhering to the treatment and accepted her 'reality' of the situation (Conn, 1993).

CHARACTERISTICS OF THE PATIENT–PHYSICIAN RELATIONSHIP

Any patient–physician encounter crosses two dimensions: instrumental and expressive (Ben-Sira, 1980; Bloom, 1963; DiMatteo and Hays, 1984). The instrumental dimension involves the physician's competence in performing the technical aspects of care, the 'science of medicine' (e.g., performing diagnostic tests and physical examinations, prescribing treatment). The expressive or affective dimension, representing the 'art of medicine', encompasses the affective components of the interaction, such as warmth and empathy, i.e., *how* the physician treats the patient. More recently, the expressive dimension has been elaborated to include both the socioemotional tone of the interaction and the clarity of communication of information between patient and physician. These two dimensions overlap to a great degree (e.g., Ben-Sira, 1980) and it is their confluence that leads to two important outcomes: adherence to recommended treatment and the patient's satisfaction with medical care. The relationships among these variables are drawn in Figure 6.1.

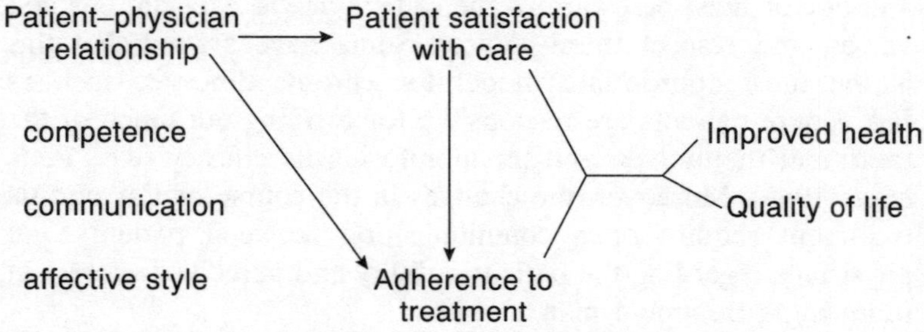

Figure 6.1 Effects of patient–physician relationship

Models of patient–physician relationships

Some would argue that the power asymmetry between patient and physician is essential to the smooth course of medical care. The patient comes in need of information or technical assistance, and the physician makes decisions that the patient must accept. While appropriate for medical emergencies, this model has lost favour in the treatment of chronic conditions, such as rheumatoid arthritis.

In a classic article that continues to have an impact four decades later, Szasz and Hollender (1956) distinguished between three models of patient–physician relationships. In all three, the relationship is a function of both the medical setting and the nature of the medical problem at hand. In the *activity–passivity* model, the physician is active and the patient passive; that is, the physician actively treats the patient, but the patient has no control, responsibility or active participation. This model is most appropriate for the treatment of medical emergencies, or when a patient is totally incapacitated or unconscious, as in the case of accidents or surgery.

The *guidance–cooperation* model is the most pervasive in current medical practice. The physician recommends a treatment and the patient cooperates with it, i.e., 'Doctor knows best'. The physician can be supportive of the patient and non-authoritarian within this model, but she assumes responsibility for deciding what treatment is appropriate. The patient is placed in a position of lesser power, and is expected to follow the physician's recommendations.

The third model, *mutual participation*, implies that patients and physicians should share responsibility for decision-making in planning, implementing and modifying treatment. Both patient and doctor must be aware of the other's needs, expectations and values, and respect these choices. Some have argued that this is the most appropriate model for chronic illnesses, such as RA, where patients are responsible for carrying out much of the treatment themselves, and for monitoring its efficacy (e.g., Potts *et al.*, 1986). Moreover, the changes in the course of RA and its treatment require open communication between patients and physicians regarding the patient's ability and perceived success in following a treatment plan.

Some rheumatologists feel that the optimal model is somewhere between guidance–cooperation and mutual participation. Some patients may be able to deal with the responsibility that the mutual-participation model implies while others cannot. The physician described earlier in Case 2, who had allowed a patient to make a medication decision (exemplifying the mutual-participation model) used the more directive guidance–cooperation model with another, older patient who had developed vasculitis (inflammation of the arteries), a serious complication of RA. The physician told the patient that he was going to increase her dosage of prednisone, and informed her of the possibility of side-effects. Although the patient was understandably concerned and suggested a less aggressive approach, and the physician thought her request reasonable, he pressured her to accept his recommendation. 'Her choices, I explained to her, were prednisone to control the process or no prednisone and possible deterioration with more disability and possibly death . . . I had made the decision based on medical knowledge I had accumulated over many years. My patient did not have that knowledge. She was not equipped to make that decision' (Conn, 1993: 25).

The character of a particular patient–physician relationship may change over time. As the patient's health status changes, so must the nature of the patient–physician relationship. With cases of long-term RA, this most often involves going from a guidance–cooperation model to a mutual-participation model. At the time of diagnosis, patient education and guidance is useful in learning how to manage symptoms. In most cases, the physician prescribes the most potentially effective treatment and the patient must cooperate with the treatment to determine its efficacy. Once treatment is stabilised, the interaction can easily move to the mutual-participation model where the patient monitors symptoms, reports problems adhering to the treatment, and works with the physician to modify the regimen and increase treatment efficacy.

Non-adherence often occurs when both patients and physicians are caught in the guidance–cooperation model. The patient may be frustrated because the treatment is not working; her pain and disability are real to her. The physician may be frustrated because she feels that the patient is not following her recommendations completely, and is not taking responsibility for her health. Both participants in this encounter are partially correct, but both need to change their behaviours and expectations toward each other and toward the relationship. When new symptoms appear or a treatment is not working despite the patient's adherence, there may be a need to temporarily shift back to the guidance–cooperation model; however, with the patient fully informed, the dyad should be able to move back to the mutual-participation model with ease.

ADHERENCE TO MEDICAL TREATMENT

Following a prescribed medical treatment plan is seen by some as the most important outcome of the patient–physician relationship and as a mediator between medical care and medical outcomes (see Figure 6.1). Patient adherence/compliance is often defined as the extent to which a patient's behaviour coincides with the therapeutic recommendation made by a health professional (DiNicola and DiMatteo, 1984). The terms cooperation, adherence and compliance have been used interchangeably in the arthritis literature. Some maintain that adherence connotes a more interactive or collaborative relationship between the patient and health care provider whereas compliance and cooperation suggest a more authoritarian relationship in which the patient is a passive responder to the physician's demands (Bradley, 1989b). Both definitions, however, imply a behavioural goal that the patient should achieve. As the term adherence implies more active and voluntary participation by the patient and is more consistent with the mutual collaboration model, it is used throughout this chapter unless a researcher's words are directly cited.

As depicted in Figure 6.1, both improved health (i.e., less pain and stiffness, slower disease progression) and quality of life are seen as the positive outcomes of adherence. The construct of quality of life has only recently been suggested as an outcome of adherence (Liang, 1989; Kaplan *et al.*, 1992). Treatments for arthritis are most often evaluated in terms of biomedical markers such as joint inflammation that reflect underlying disease processes. These are seldom evaluated for their effects on functional and psychological well-being, described in Chapter 4 as the core components of quality of life.

The effectiveness of most RA treatment is dependent on patients' carrying out treatment recommendations, which often involve taking oral medication, exercising and wearing splints. Treatment may also involve lifestyle changes (e.g., changing diet or work habits) or keeping regularly scheduled appointments for medical check-ups or physical or occupational therapy. Agras has written that 'a breakdown of behaviour at any one of these levels will deleteriously affect compliance and outcome of treatment' (1989, p. S2). There are a number of underlying assumptions in this statement. The first involves the definition and measurement of adherence; the second implies a belief that the treatment is appropriate and effective; the third involves the association of a behaviour (adherence) with an outcome (improved health); and the fourth that the patient is able (or believes she is able) to carry out the treatment plan.

The first assumption involves the definitions of adherence and non-adherence. Is non-adherence the complete failure to follow prescribed treatment? If a patient is advised to take a particular medication, perform exercises at home, and wear a splint at night, is she not cooperating if she omits any one of these components? Or if she takes less than the prescribed dosage of medication? What if she takes the prescribed dosage, but at irregular intervals? Or takes *more* than the prescribed dosage? Is this patient non-adherent if she follows all three prescribed recommendations to the letter, but also adopts an unproven remedy, such as wearing a copper bracelet, praying daily, or taking a dietary supplement?

The underlying question is whether these variations have equally serious health consequences. When does non-adherence matter? How much adherence is necessary for a given therapy to be effective (Deyo, 1982)? Adherence is not a dichotomous variable with patients characterised as adherent or not, but ranges along a number of continua related to the nature of the treatment regimen. Most patients are neither good nor bad adherers in an absolute sense, but may adhere perfectly to one aspect of the treatment regimen while ignoring another, or adhere at one time and not another. Liang (1989) argues that non-compliance is a more complex phenomenon than simply deviant behaviour and that it can only be addressed within the context of the person's life-goals and quality of life with and without the treatment.

Patients may complement physicians' recommendations with unproven or non-traditional treatments. Is this non-adherence? In a large random sample of a Western US community survey, 84 per cent of respondents with a musculoskeletal disorder used one or more unconventional remedies (Cronan *et al.*, 1989). Behavioural/cognitive remedies, such as prayer, relaxation therapy, bedrest, (non-prescribed) exercise, and massage were used most often, and were perceived to be the most effective. Exotic remedies such as copper bracelets or dietary remedies were used by only a small proportion of the subjects, and were not perceived as effective. The authors of the study suggest that most unconventional remedies are not harmful and appear to have subjective benefits, providing patients with a sense of control over their illness.

A second assumption is that the treatment has been accurately prescribed and is effective. This assumption must be held by both physician and patient. For example, pharmacologic agents are prescribed with the assumption that they will do more than relieve symptoms; they will alter the natural progression of the disease in some way. However, research suggests that pharmacologic treatment for rheumatoid arthritis may have only short-term gains and may not delimit future morbidity (Weisman, 1989). Moreover, there is considerable disagreement as to what types of treatment are most effective for RA, particularly in the early years (Wilske and Healy, 1989).

Patients' doubts regarding the value of treatment may lead to non-adherence. Agras has argued that 'patients should not be expected to comply with ineffective or mismanaged treatments' (Agras 1989, p. S2). This type of non-adherence has been termed 'rational noncompliance' (Becker, 1985), but is still framed as a deviant behaviour, maintaining the emphasis on the patient's motivated refusal to adhere to treatment.

A third assumption is that behavioural adherence to a prescribed treatment will lead to a desired health outcome, such as pain reduction, increased mobility, or slower progression of the disease. This assumed relationship between behaviour and outcome is important for understanding non-adherence for two reasons. First, if patients are following the treatment plan and see little or no improvement, this outcome may lead them to lapse in the behaviour, as they do not perceive their actions as being effective. Some patients stop following the treatment plan when they do not perceive a net health benefit or when the costs outweigh the benefits, for example in the case of uncomfortable or disabling side-effects. Second, the lack of a connection between what they do and what the outcome is may colour patients' beliefs more generally about the efficacy of treatment, leading to reduced adherence later on. Even perfect behavioural adherence may not result in improved health (Kaplan *et al.*, 1989). From his personal experience, Liang (1989), a rheumatologist, describes the most frequently given reasons for treatment non-adherence as 'Didn't work' and 'Worked only a little while'.

The fourth assumption involves self-efficacy beliefs, that the patient believes she is capable of initiating and continuing to follow the treatment. Patients feel less able to carry out treatment when it is complex or when it interferes with daily routines (Bradley, 1989b). Thus, treatments which are simplified, for example, daily medication in one dosage instead of multiple administrations, or exercises that can be fitted into one's schedule increase self-efficacy beliefs as patients experience more initial success.

Estimates of adherence to RA treatment

Although adherence behaviour among RA patients has been studied primarily in terms of medication usage, research has also examined home exercise, splint usage, physical therapy, and self-management of pain as outcomes. Reviews of the literature among adult RA patients suggest that adherence with medication regimens ranges from 30 per cent to 78 per cent (Bradley, 1989b; Deyo, 1982; Liang, 1989). This range is similar to rates of non-adherence for all diseases, including conditions more asymptomatic than RA (15 per cent to 93 per cent; Kaplan *et al.*, 1993). Rates of non-adherence for exercise have been found to be equivalent to or higher than those for oral medication, from 34 per cent to 62 per cent (Bradley, 1989b; Liang, 1989).

The wide range of reported adherence reflects not only individual differences, but also lack of precision in its measurement. Self-reports have been the most commonly used measurement technique in studies of arthritis (Dunbar *et al.*, 1989). However, patient self-reports may be inaccurate because of a reliance on memory or an inability to self-monitor. It has also been suggested that patients' reports of adherence are often positively biased because of expectations and a desire to please the physician or one's family, but the empirical evidence is equivocal. Although Oakes *et al.* (1970) found a direct relationship between patients' use of splints and their perceptions of whether family members expected them to wear the splint, Moon *et al.* (1976) found no association between patients' perceptions of their physician's expectations of compliance and wearing a hand splint.

Estimates of adherence vary with the type of treatment recommended. For example self-reports of oral medication often provide higher estimates than more objective measures such as return pill counts, medication refills, or blood serum pharmacologic markers (Bradley, 1989b; Deyo *et al.*, 1981; Dunbar *et al.*, 1989). Physicians seem to be no better than patients in estimating adherence; physicians or allied health care providers overestimate the extent to which their patients adhere to prescribed treatment (DiMatteo and DiNicola, 1982; Geersten *et al.*, 1973; Lee and Tan,

1979; Moon *et al.*, 1976). Inaccuracies also may originate in physicians' refusals to acknowledge non-adherence in their patients and to discuss this with their patients. Direct questions regarding patients' behaviour are rarely asked in the typical patient–physician encounter (DiNicola and DiMatteo, 1984).

Factors affecting adherence

Research has identified a host of risk factors for non-adherence to treatment for RA and other chronic illnesses, such as characteristics of the treatment regimen (e.g., duration or complexity, the extent of side-effects), characteristics of the patient (e.g., age, social class, beliefs about treatment efficacy), characteristics of the patient's social setting (e.g., family support), and influences of the health care setting (Agras, 1989). It is the latter set of factors that are the focus for the remainder of this chapter. There have been a number of excellent reviews of the literature pertaining to adherence to RA treatment for adults (Belcon *et al.*, 1984; Bradley, 1989b; Deyo, 1982a; Feinberg, 1988) and children (Rapoff, 1989), and in clinical trials (Deyo, 1982; Probstfield, 1989). Other reviews focus on techniques for improving patient adherence (Jette, 1982; Daltroy, 1993; Hovell and Black, 1989). As the purpose of this chapter is not to review the entire literature on adherence to RA treatment, the reader is referred to those other sources for a complete and detailed discussion of the issues.

The quality of the patient–provider relationship appears to be an especially important determinant of adherence. Two aspects of the patient–physician relationship will be discussed: communication, particularly the provision of information, and affective style. In addition, satisfaction with care, which is related to both the communicative and affective qualities of the patient–physician relationship, will be discussed as it serves as a mediating variable between the patient–physician relationship and adherence to treatment (as shown in Figure 6.1).

Patient–physician communication and adherence

Patient–physician communication may be the single most important variable affecting adherence (e.g., Bradley, 1989b). The issue of communication must be seen within a dyadic interactional framework involving two actors. For successful communication the physician must present information clearly while the patient needs to seek clarification and ensure that her concerns are addressed. In one study, learning how to communicate with the doctor was rated by RA patients as their primary educational need (Buckley *et al.*, 1990), and for every educational and psychosocial need named, patients rated their physician as first choice to provide that information (in preference to education groups and individual counsellors). There is no doubt that patients look to their physicians for guidance, information and comfort across a wide range of medical and non-medical issues.

The provision of information necessary for managing one's arthritis and following the treatment plan is the central component of the patient–physician encounter for chronic conditions. DiNicola and DiMatteo (1984) refer to this as the *instructional* component of communication. As Daltroy states with elegant simplicity (1993: 224), 'patients are not active in seeking information and physicians are not active in giving it'. This may occur because of the time constraints of most medical visits, impersonal health care environments, the inequity in power and status residing with the patient–physician encounter, patients' unfamiliarity with medical language or physicians' inability to enter the patient's perspective. Physicians often underestimate how much information patients desire, and patients often fail to inform the physician when they do not understand the information presented. An example of such a misunderstanding to communicate occurred with a patient who woke himself in the middle of the night because his doctor had told him to take his medication four times over a 24-hour period, despite the fact that his broken sleep was contributing to his fatigue. When asked why he had not contacted his physician about this, he countered, 'Why would the doctor have gone to the trouble of telling me that it was to be taken over a 24-hour period?' As this example shows, information about how to carry out the prescribed treatment must be presented clearly and simply for it to be understood. Even if the information is presented clearly, however, in both spoken and written form, patients may not understand it or may interpret it differently.

A number of factors may thwart patient–physician communication. First and foremost is the clarity of the explanation concerning the diagnosis and the course and purpose of treatment. In a study of drug compliance in RA, a higher proportion of compliant (53 per cent) vs non-compliant patients (31 per cent) felt that they had received an adequate explanation of their illness (Lee and Tan, 1979). In another study, arthritis patients questioned several days after a medical visit did not understand the purpose of 15 per cent of their prescriptions (Daltroy, 1993). Four months later, these patients had compliance rates twice as high for the prescriptions whose purpose they had understood (58 per cent vs 29 per cent). A second study confirmed the importance of understanding the purpose of medications: when rheumatologists were recorded as having made a clear statement about the purpose of a drug, 79 per cent of the patients were compliant 4 months later in comparison to only 33 per cent when the rheumatologist's statement was not clear (Daltroy, 1993). Patients must understand the purpose of the treatment and the exact steps they will need to take to carry it out in order to achieve even a semblance of adherence.

Physicians have beliefs about what and how much information should be provided. Some believe that patients are laypersons who cannot understand the processes underlying their disease or the mechanisms underlying treatment. For some groups of patients this becomes even more salient – for example, aged patients (Haug and Ory, 1987), patients with little education, or patients from a different culture or who speak a different language (Seijo *et al.*, 1991). These assumptions may not be totally unwarranted. Some older patients do exhibit forgetfulness and a lack of concentration or recall, or are unable or unwilling to express their deepest concerns (Haug and Ory, 1987). When patients and physicians do not communicate in the same language and/or come from different cultures, mutual understanding is reduced (Seijo *et al.*, 1991). Physicians vary widely in their ability to listen to the patient or to understand the 'subtext' of their expressed concerns. Asking only specific, closed questions may not lead to the crucial problem and may lead to a premature formulation of a diagnosis or treatment plan.

Ineffective communication may also result in the over-use of medical jargon and technical language. Physicians use jargon in talking to other professionals, and this natural way of speaking in medical settings often carries over in conversations with patients. Alternately, use of jargon can symbolise a withholding of information and an explicit attempt to exert authority over a patient. Whatever the cause, medical jargon often leads to a failure to comprehend or a distortion of what has been said.

Communication also may be impaired when the patient and physician hold different beliefs about the illness and its treatment. Patients are likely to follow treatment if they believe in its efficacy. For example, in a study conducted by Arluke (1980), some RA patients held the belief that a drug's efficacy would decrease over time, and stopped their medication at the first sign of improvement.

Patients' health beliefs, values and expectations are potent factors affecting adherence, not only because of their direct relationship to health behaviour, but also because they are subject to misinterpretation by physicians and likely to influence how satisfied patients will be with the consultation. Several studies have shown that physicians misperceive their patients' desires regarding the amount, content, and preferred method for providing information on arthritis and its treatments (Lorig *et al.*, 1984; Potts *et al.*, 1984).

Because RA is a chronic illness, many patients will have had considerable experience with the health care system, with different providers and, often, a long-term relationship with a single rheumatologist. Many will have experienced a number of treatment modalities, from pharmacologic interventions to physical therapy to splints. Many will be quite knowledgeable about their disease, and may have more sophisticated perceptions about the effectiveness of treatments and the advisability of changing protocols than physicians appreciate. At the same time, arthritis patients with longer-term disease, lower physical functioning and greater depression have been shown to have lower expectations for the efficacy of their treatment (Ross *et al.*, 1990), which may lead to lower adherence.

Physician's affective style and adherence

In addition to the instructional component, discussed above, DiNicola and DiMatteo (1984) describe a second component of patient–physician communication that affects adherence: the physician's affective style. Perceptions of physician friendliness, caring, warmth, sensitivity, concern, interest and respect are the ingredients of patient–physician rapport. These may derive from the actual exchange between doctor and patient, or be reflected in more structural factors such as excessive waiting times, inconvenient hours and brief encounters.

Geersten *et al.* (1973) found that long waits were related to both dissatisfaction with medical care and lower rates of compliance among RA patients (as estimated by the physician). Patients who felt that the physician spent adequate time with them and was more personable (as opposed to business-like), and who rated patient–physician communication as better, had higher rates of compliance. The interrelated effects of these variables lend support to the model depicted in Figure 6.1.

Non-verbal behaviour can be of great importance in the communication of warmth and caring to patients (DiMatteo and Hays, 1984; Friedman, 1982). Patients have a great sensitivity to non-verbal communication such as facial expressions, voice tones, gestures and touch. Warmth and caring can be conveyed through eye contact, open arm positions, smiling, head nodding and touch. Research examining gaze has shown that a physician's refusal to look a patient directly in the eye leads to difficulties establishing rapport. The tone of voice transmits expectancies and authority. The process is bidirectional so that the non-verbal expressiveness by the patient provides cues that the physician will interpret and respond to.

Patients' sensitivity to physicians' non-verbal behaviour has been linked to satisfaction with care and choosing one physician over another. Physicians' sensitivity to patients' non-verbal cues may suggest empathy and promote adherence; for example, listening shows that the physician respects the patient (Stiles *et al.*, 1979).

In most cases non-verbal communication reinforces the spoken word; at times, however, it may contradict or complement what the physician is saying. In a study of patient–physician conversations, Hall *et al.* (1981) found that physicians' positive statements in combination with a negative affective tone in their voice was most strongly linked with patient satisfaction, reflecting both warmth *and* concern.

Satisfaction with care

Patient satisfaction is an important outcome of medical care itself, but also may be a critical determinant of the decision to adhere to a prescribed treatment, or even to continue medical care. Most of the empirical literature on satisfaction with medical care deals with single first-visit encounters among patients with undiagnosed symptoms or acute illness in primary care clinics. Less research has been conducted on long-term patient–physician relationships or care for chronic illnesses such as RA, making it difficult to know whether the research findings can be directly applied to arthritis populations.

Overall, there are three dimensions along which satisfaction with the doctor–patient relationship can be considered: satisfaction with the amount and quality of the information provided by the doctor (informational satisfaction); the extent to which the patient feels that the doctor listens, understands and is interested (interpersonal or affective satisfaction); and the patient's evaluation of the doctor's competence (technical satisfaction). In several studies, Ben-Sira (1980, 1985) found strong associations between patients' evaluations of the technical and interpersonal aspects of their care. Stiles *et al.* (1979) reported that affective satisfaction was associated with the amount of time during the visit in which the *patient* gave information to the doctor (explaining the problem in their own words); in contrast, informational satisfaction was related to the amount of time that the *physician* spent giving information to the patient.

Some research has suggested that satisfaction is a proxy for the physician's ability to communicate concern, warmth and interest. When the physician addresses the patient's concerns during a visit, satisfaction with care increases (Ben-Sira, 1976; DiMatteo and Hays, 1984). For example, among RA patients with long-term disease, those who indicated that their concerns had been reduced during a medical visit were more satisfied with the care they received (Potts *et al.*, 1986).

Physicians may not elicit or discuss psychosocial concerns because they believe they are irrelevant, time-consuming, and/or outside of their expertise (Daltroy, 1993), or because they have difficulty knowing how to respond to these concerns. This is a particularly important issue with respect to care of the elderly. Older people are more likely to have experienced social losses, such as deaths of significant others, that may affect their emotional state and motivation to continue treatment. Psychological distress may be somatised, by the exaggeration of physical symptoms, while emotional symptoms remain masked. Unfortunately, virtually no research has addressed physicians' perceptions of their role as providers of socioemotional support.

THE INFLUENCE OF AGE AND GENDER ON THE PHYSICIAN–PATIENT RELATIONSHIP

In most studies of doctor–patient relationships, the gender of the physician, and often of the patient as well, is ignored. The unstated assumption is that the genders of the patient and physician do not influence their interaction. Indeed, in Western medicine, most physicians *have* been men. But as more women enter medicine, the gender of the physician becomes a salient factor in evaluating the quality of the physician–patient relationship, particularly along the affective dimensions of care (Miles, 1991). Similarly, the social demography of RA indicates that most patients with RA are female, and many, particularly those with long-term illness, are older women. Thus, a brief discussion of the issues of age and gender as they influence the patient–physician relationship is warranted.

There is evidence that the genders of the patient and the physician have an effect on the patient–physician relationship and its outcomes. Similarly, there is research suggesting that the age of the patient may shape encounters and treatment decisions. Most of this research is not in the area of rheumatology, but in general practice. This section concentrates on two issues: the attitudes of physicians towards women patients and older patients, and differences between men and women physicians as they affect the patient–physician relationship.

The age of the patient

The age of the patient may impinge on patient–provider relationships in a number of ways. Many difficulties in following a treatment regimen or communicating with physicians are rooted in older peoples' social situations and health beliefs, and require sensitivity on the part of the physician (Haug and Ory, 1987). For example, the sensory losses associated with ageing, such as visual or hearing losses, may impair the ability to understand the details of the treatment regimen. Complex pharmaceutical regimens, often the case for older people with multiple chronic illnesses, may be confusing to follow.

Health care practitioners, researchers and patients alike have expressed concern about the extent to which health care professionals' attitudes and beliefs lead them to use age as a cue for making treatment decisions. Medical students receive little training in geriatrics, and negative attitudes toward the elderly have been documented among first-year medical students (Spence *et al.*, 1968), hospital house staff (Solomon and Vickers, 1979), and other health care professionals (Baker, 1984; Cilberto *et al.*, 1981). Medical staff spend less time with older patients (Keeler *et al.*, 1982), treat their symptoms less aggressively (Kvitek *et al.*, 1986), and respond less to their psychosocial concerns (Greene *et al.*, 1987). These behaviours, in turn, may decrease patient satisfaction and increase unwillingness to seek or continue needed treatment (Nuttbrock and Kosberg, 1980).

A number of studies have examined the effect of age stereotypes on the attitudes and behaviours of physicians or other health care professionals. Stereotypes, quite simply, are cognitive short-cuts that guide how people take in, remember, and make inferences about information they process. In the absence of specific information about a particular individual, people rely on generalised beliefs about a group the individual belongs to – for example, old people – to make judgements and decisions. Often these generalised beliefs are not accurate when applied to that particular individual and can often become fixed as prejudices.

Two studies of physicians' use of stereotypes with rheumatoid arthritis patients have been conducted by Revenson and her colleagues. Using an experimental methodology, Revenson (1989) examined the influence of age stereotypes on rheumatologists' attitudes and behavioural intentions to provide information and social support to RA patients depicted in case histories. It was predicted that increased contact with older patients (operationalised as a greater proportion of patients over 65 in their practice) would decrease physicians' reliance on stereotypes and increase perceptions of individual attributes. Rheumatologists in the study were presented with one of two identical case histories of a female RA patient, only in one condition the target patient was age 53 and in the other was 83. Contrary to predictions, the more contact physicians had with elderly patients, the more they tended to use stereotypes. However, these stereotypes were not negative evaluations of the older patient, but what has been termed *compassionate stereotypes* (Binstock, 1983) that showed concern for the older patients because of infirmities and helplessness. However, it was not clear whether the rheumatologists' ratings were based on age *per se* or assumptions about the level of disability for the age group.

In a second study using a similar methodology but including case histories of both male and female target patients and controlling for level of disability, Revenson and colleagues (1992) found that physicians again made differential ratings on the basis of the patient's age, such that a 73-year-old target was seen as more instrumental, autonomous and well-adjusted than a 43-year-old. Whether the target patient was a man or a woman did not affect physicians' ratings. Because all patients in the case histories were portrayed as being employed part-time (to control level of disability), the older patients may have been seen as less disabled because they were more atypical for their age group. In fact, physicians did rate the older targets as less typical patients for their age than the younger targets, though they were rated as no less disabled. This finding may reflect a more subtle influence of age stereotypes on physicians' attitudes.

The influence of gender on age stereotypes has received relatively little research attention, although patient gender has been shown to be relevant to the course and content of interactions between elderly patients and physicians (Haug and Ory, 1987). Gender stereotypes may become less pronounced as individuals age, because they are replaced with ageing stereotypes (Revenson *et al.*, 1992). Alternately, there may be a 'double standard' of ageing that puts older women at a disadvantage because they are members of two stereotyped groups (Sontag, 1979). The physical appearance that accompanies ageing is more acceptable among men than women, leading to more negative evaluations of women. This double standard may be especially pronounced among older women with rheumatoid arthritis because of visible disability, e.g. deformed hands or feet. For older women, who are already stereotyped as more passive and dependent than older men or younger women, the disability stereotype may act to reinforce the negative images of unattractiveness, dependency, and low worth.

The gender of the patient

Research suggests that gender may affect the nature and quality of medical treatment for a variety of diseases. For example, recent evidence has been presented showing that the aggressiveness and type of treatment for coronary heart disease differs for women and men (Wenger, 1990), and that men receive more expensive medical check-ups than women across a variety of illnesses (Armitage *et al.*, 1979). There is also a substantial literature gathered over the past two decades that sex stereotypes may affect definitions of mental health and treatment decisions for psychological problems (Travis, 1988; Pilgrim and Rogers, 1983).

A number of studies suggest that physicians' sex-role stereotypes may bias their assessments of women's medical complaints (Verbrugge and Steiner, 1984). Specifically, physicians tend to see female patients as more emotional and making excessive demands (Bernstein and Kane, 1981; Colameco *et al.*, 1983), to take women's medical complaints less seriously (Armitage *et al.*, 1979) and to classify their conditions as less serious (Verbrugge, 1980), frequently attributing them to psychosomatic causes (e.g., Armitage *et al.*, 1979; Bernstein and Kane, 1979; Wallen *et al.*, 1979). Wallen *et al.* (1979) tape-recorded interactions between male physicians and their male and female patients and found that physicians discouraged communication and information exchange more often with female than with male patients. However, it is interesting that these gender differences do not appear or are less pronounced in experimental studies using hypothetical cases (Colameco *et al.*, 1983; McCrainie *et al.* 1978; Revenson *et al.*, 1992). It is possible that experimental methods may not be suited to studying dyadic interaction, and that 'real' patients elicit affective responses and/or sex-role stereotypes from their physicians.

With the exception of the studies conducted by Revenson, there have been no studies of gender stereotyping among practitioners treating people with RA. Possibly, because RA is more prevalent among women, physicians expect to see more women with RA in their practice, and take their physical complaints more seriously. In addition, there is such within-gender variability that physicians may be able to contrast patients without respect to gender. Rheumatologists also may take women's emotional concerns more seriously because they are aware of the stress of adhering to the treatment regimen over a long period and are likely to have developed a rapport with patients over the course of the illness. There is, however, some indication that gender stereotypes continue to be invoked with fibromyalgia syndrome: recent studies indicate that (female) patients are often told that their symptoms are imagined or psychogenic in origin (Goldenberg, 1987).

The gender of the physician

The increase in the number of women physicians in the past 20 years has led to research exploring whether and how women physicians relate differently to patients, and whether these differences affect medical care (see review by Martin, Arnold, *et al.*, 1988). If the gender of the physician *does* affect the patient–physician relationship, it is likely to do so through a number of the key dimensions discussed earlier in the chapter: physicians' attitudes and expectations; communication of information between doctor and patient; and the affective tone of the relationship (Waller, 1988).

The general perception is that women physicians are more humanistic and empathic than their male colleagues, but the limited research in this area does not offer any conclusive evidence. As a result of their socialisation, female physicians may have different values and ideological views from those held by their male colleagues. They also may view women's roles and behaviours in a different light. Their interpersonal skills affecting their interactions with patients and, consequently, their medical decisions, may be different from those of male physicians. At the same time, believing that women physicians are more empathic, patients disclose more symptoms or psychosocial issues affecting adherence. Gender also may have an effect on the power differentials between patient and physician (Lorber, 1987), with female physicians being less assertive or being perceived as less powerful by the patient.

Studies have failed to uncover gender differences in technical or diagnostic skills, or in general attitudes toward patient care (Martin, Arnold, *et al.*, 1988); for example, there is little evidence that women medical students are more nurturant than men or have more patient-oriented attitudes (McGrath and Zimet, 1977) or that women and men internists hold different attitudes toward patients (Colameco *et al.*, 1983). A number of studies, however, show strong gender differences in communication and practice styles (Martin, Arnold, *et al.*, 1988). Women doctors spend more time with patients than do men (e.g., Bensing *et al.*, 1993; Roter *et al.*, 1991), and engage in more conversation during a medical visit (Roter *et al.*, 1991). Specifically, they engage in more positive talk, partnership building, and question-asking, and provide more medical and psychosocial information (Roter *et al.*, 1991).

Observing doctor–patient interaction in a sample of general-practice residents, Shapiro (1990) found that women physicians outperformed males in areas such as responding to patients' non-verbal cues, requesting psychosocial information from patients, consulting with others, looking up information and discussing the psychosocial impact of the disease on patient and family.

These studies suggest that women doctors may be more skilful at communicating with patients and in developing rapport. Consequently, they may be better able to listen and elicit salient information than are men doctors. West's deconstructions of patient–physician conversations (1993) revealed that men physicians interrupted patients more frequently than women physicians, whereas women physicians interrupted their patients as frequently as they were interrupted by the patients. Interruptions not only interfere with patients' expositions of their symptoms and health status, but may also undercut confidence and trust in the physician.

There is also evidence that women physicians may be more willing than men physicians to form egalitarian relationships with patients (Miles, 1991; Weisman and Teitelbaum, 1985). This is especially true for women doctors treating women: women doctors, who have broken sex-role stereotypes themselves, may be less likely to assume that women are passive by nature and need decisions to be made for them. Greene *et al.* (1987), studying internal medicine residents and older patients, observed that women physicians were more egalitarian in their interactions with patients, more responsive to patients' psychosocial issues, and more respectful of their concerns. If a non-authoritarian attitude fosters rapport with elderly patients, then women physicians may have an advantage.

Several studies have found that patients hold an image of women physicians as more empathic and better listeners (Martin, Arnold, *et al.*, 1988). In one study of patient satisfaction with internal medicine residents (Comstock *et al.*, 1982), women patients seeing women physicians expressed greater satisfaction with their care than did any other dyad.

Whether women and men physicians do relate to patients differently, and, more importantly, whether these differences affect medical care remain open questions. There is relatively little research on actual patient–physician interactions, and none within the specialty of rheumatology and musculoskeletal disease. Thus, generalisations are made from studies of internal medicine and family practice. Moreover, research examining differences between female and male physicians has not examined the influence of gender socialisation on physicians or the influences of medical socialisation, which might smooth out (Leserman, 1981) *or* accentuate these differences (West, 1993).

IMPROVING PATIENT–PHYSICIAN RELATIONSHIPS

The literature reviewed in this chapter has demonstrated that both the informational and affective components of communication affect patient satisfaction and adherence behaviour. Although it is questionable whether doctors can be taught to become empathic beings (Sarason, 1985) or whether patients can be taught to be highly informed health care consumers during a very stressful time in their lives, psychological theory and research provide a number of means by which more honest, open and transactional patient–physician relationships can be achieved.

One alternative was to end this chapter with suggestions on 'what the doctor can do' and 'what the patient can do'. This reinforces a separateness of patient and physician that contradicts the conceptual framework presented here of the patient–physician interaction as a transactional process. Instead, Daltroy's (1993) recommendations for improving patient–physician encounters are presented because they assign responsibility to both patients and physicians and focus on the transaction and not the players.

In an excellent chapter on doctor–patient communication in rheumatological disorders, Daltroy (1993) has described nine tasks that must be met during a physician–patient encounter in order to achieve a balanced flow of communication and a trusting relationship. These tasks are listed in Table 6.1. The tasks focus directly on improving communication in the patient–physician relationship, for example having the doctor and patient share their goals for treatment. This approach capitalises on the fact that patient–physician relationships in chronic illness unfold over time. The focus of patient–physician encounters changes as the core task shifts from identifying initial symptoms and complaints to diagnosis to discussing and implementing treatment to modifying treatment based on symptom changes, new concerns, treatment efficacy and the patient's lifestyle.

Table 6.1 Tasks of patient–physician communication

1	The patient expresses all his or her concerns during the medical encounter
2	The doctor addresses all the patient's concerns
3	Doctor and patient share models of disease and symptoms
4	Doctor and patient share goals for treatment
5	Doctor and patient agree on treatment goals and set priorities
6	Doctor and patient share models of treatment
7	Doctor and patient identify potential compliance difficulties
8	Doctor and patient plan how to overcome anticipated compliance difficulties
9	The doctor provides written information on the disease and the treatment regimen

Source: Daltroy (1993: 230–4)

Most of the tasks are pertinent to or directly address the issue of adherence to treatment, a central component of arthritis care. Daltroy also lists twelve specific techniques that physicians can use (1993: 235). For example, he suggests that both the doctor and the patient identify potential compliance difficulties and jointly plan how to overcome them. Once these concerns are 'on the table' the physician can suggest changes in the regimen that might facilitate adherence, and the patient can think through changes in her lifestyle that might increase adherence. Thus, both patient and physician employ anticipatory instrumental coping. The physician might suggest coping strategies that other patients have used successfully and patients might plan ways to include family members in the treatment plan, providing themselves with social support and coping assistance.

Although physicians are allowed to use their greater medical knowledge in these encounters, the nine tasks exemplify Szasz and Hollender's (1956) model of mutual participation. In fact, the nine tasks almost constitute a covenant between physician and patient. This approach holds great promise for improving medical care and has the potential to be developed into a structured intervention for use in medical education. More specific suggestions for how to implement these tasks are provided in Daltroy (1993: 230–4).

Although Daltroy's task-focused framework directly tackles the issue of patient–physician communication with strategies that can be implemented easily, it provides no substantive advice for improving the affective quality of the patient–physician relationship. Research indicates that the affective style of the physician is often judged by patients to be the crucial component of satisfaction with medical care (Ben-Sira, 1980, 1985). While it is questionable whether doctors, or more accurately medical students, can be taught compassion and humility (Sarason, 1985), medical education can and has used strategies to train physicians to be more aware of the verbal and non-verbal cues they transmit, and to be more sensitive to cues sent by patients. Similarly, the teaching of effective communication on the lay side of the patient–physician transaction may be useful for patients negotiating the medical system (Hall *et al.*, 1981).

Speedling and Rose (1985) have suggested that interventions aimed at improving the patient–physician relationship (and ultimately adherence and health outcomes) move from a goal of increasing patient satisfaction to increasing patient *participation*. Echoing the mutual participation model of Szasz and Hollender proposed 30 years earlier, Speedling and Rose suggest that physicians encourage patients to take an active role in decision-making and management of health problems. This does not mean that physicians should take a more passive role, but that physicians minimise their use of coercive power and maximise their use of expert power (knowledge) and referent power (modelling) (Rodin and Janis, 1982), empowering patients in their own treatment.

SUMMARY

This chapter has focused on two areas: the process of patient–physician interactions, which involves communication, and the outcome of these interactions, in terms of adherence to treatment and satisfaction with care. It has been found that expressions of warmth, personal concern and interest, and the provision of understandable information and suggestions, appear to be strongly related to both patient satisfaction and adherence.

Chapter 7

Coping with rheumatoid arthritis

INTRODUCTION

The range of issues that present themselves to someone with rheumatoid arthritis have been well documented in earlier chapters. We have described how pain, stiffness and disability are the major effects of the illness that have to be dealt with in some way. But the effects of RA spread much more widely than the direct symptoms of the disease (Meenan *et al.*, 1981). For example, the impact of RA disability is more wide-ranging than simply restrictions in movement. Having one's mobility reduced limits the possibilities of employment and, in turn, income. Being restricted in mobility and income in turn limit the ability to engage in pleasurable leisure and social activities as well as in maintaining roles such as breadwinner, or childrearer. Financial restrictions limit the possibilities of obtaining medical or other assistance over and above that provided by the state or insurance. Moreover, because RA has a variable course, it is not predictable and the uncertainty that this creates requires some adjustment and creates difficulties of its own (see Chapter 2). One of the difficulties of studying the ways in which individuals adapt to arthritis is this widespread impact of the disease and the disabilities which often accompany it.

Research regarding the way in which individuals cope with rheumatoid arthritis has been growing in recent years (see review by Zautra and Manne, 1992). This body of work may be divided into studies that have examined coping with rheumatoid arthritis in general and those that have focused on coping with specific symptoms of RA, such as pain. Both approaches will be discussed in this chapter. Many of the more general studies have used a methodology in which patients describe their coping efforts with regard to the stressor that affects them most. A few studies have focused on the widespread impact of RA. In evaluating these studies to gain a better understanding of the coping process, it is important to be clear as to exactly which aspects of RA the individual is trying to cope with.

CONCEPTUAL ISSUES IN COPING

The concept of coping has been embraced by individuals of different theoretical persuasions. Early work adopted a psychodynamic approach, in which coping was assessed by means of a clinical interview and *a priori* assumptions were made as to which forms of coping were adaptive (Haan, 1977; Vaillant, 1977). Within this approach, coping was viewed as synonymous with (good) adaptation according to a predetermined criterion; for example, the use of denial as a coping strategy was considered to lead to poor psychological well-being. This work had limited appeal to those who did not subscribe to psychodynamic theory (Stone *et al.*, 1992). Other researchers attempted to build on this early work to develop questionnaires to assess what they felt were dispositional approaches to coping. These not only assumed a consistency of coping efforts across situations but were also prescriptive in designating certain coping strategies as adaptive. Later researchers broke away from dynamic theory and developed relatively short self-report questionnaires to assess coping efforts in response to stress. These developments opened the way for the considerable growth in coping research over the 1980s and 1990s.

The most frequently applied approach from this later trend of research is the transactional stress and coping paradigm laid out by Lazarus and Folkman (Lazarus and Folkman, 1984; Lazarus, 1993). The transactional model has two central components. The first involves cognitive appraisals: an appraisal to evaluate the situation or stressful encounter (primary appraisal) and an appraisal of what can be done about it (secondary appraisal). The second component of the transactional model is *coping*, defined as 'ongoing cognitive and behavioural efforts to manage specific external and/or internal demands' (Lazarus 1993: 237). This conceptual approach spawned a self-report measure, the Ways of Coping questionnaire (WOC: Folkman and Lazarus 1980, 1988) which has been used or adapted in many studies of RA. The technique for assessing coping embodies a number of principles which raise important conceptual and practical issues in any examination of coping with RA.

A fundamental issue in the conceptualisation of coping is whether coping is seen as a conscious or unconscious process. Within health psychology, coping is typically seen as a conscious attempt to deal with an external stressor (Folkman and Lazarus, 1980). By this approach coping techniques could be revealed by questionnaires. A very different approach has been adopted by those who view coping as some form of defence mechanism. For the latter, coping is seen as an unconscious process which is revealed by a clinician and/or some form of projective testing. This basic distinction between conscious or purposeful processes and unconscious processes reflects the different theoretical positions underlying these approaches. The polarisation between conscious/purposeful coping and unconscious coping ignores the importance of considering coping strategies to be on a dimension of purposefulness. For example 'wishful thinking' appears to be of an order of purposefulness somewhat different to seeking social support (Newman, 1990; Zautra and Manne, 1992). It would also not be unreasonable to consider some forms of coping as habitual responses which may or may not have had an earlier conscious rationale (Newman, 1990).

Another issue is whether coping is seen as a stable or dynamic entity. This issue has frequently been framed as whether coping should be viewed as a personality (or personality-based) variable, that is, a disposition which does not change substantially over time, or whether it should be considered as a cognitive or behavioural response to a stressful situation which is subject to change as it is influenced by the context. The transactional approach (Lazarus and Folkman, 1984) defines coping as a dynamic process. Coping is seen as a constantly changing phenomenon that is both situation and outcome specific. The cognitive appraisal of a situation as stressful (i.e., posing threat, harm/loss, or challenge) leads to coping efforts which in turn modify appraisals. Thus any assessment of coping at a particular point in time will be immediately out-of-date in relation to the individual's psychological state, as by this theory, the act of coping will have led to a reappraisal of the situation (and thus to different implications for subsequent coping efforts). The assessment of coping within a transactional approach, therefore, does not make possible an independent consideration of how appraisal and coping interact (see also Stone *et al.*, 1992).

While most researchers using the WOC inventory (and thus the transactional model) have asked individuals to focus on a specific event, some have elicited responses to how individuals 'generally behave' – those studying RA, how they behave in relation to their illness. Dealing with an acute stressor, such as impending surgery, is a more specific and time-limited event than dealing with a chronic stressor, for example, lifelong illness. The issue of change over time, as the illness progresses through symptoms flares, periods of remission or steady declines in function imply that the amount of stress confronted by a person with RA will not be constant. In addition there is a daily temporal feature of RA unlike other illnesses, where morning stiffness dissipates and pain and fatigue arise throughout the day whilst performing certain tasks. It is issues such as these that make the study of coping with a chronic illness a significantly greater challenge to understand than coping with a discrete, time-limited stressful event (Pearlin and Schooler, 1978).

MODES OF COPING

The recent approaches to coping, originating with the transactional model (Lazarus and Folkman, 1984) have been dominated by the distinction between *emotion-focused* and *problem-focused* modes of coping. Problem-focused coping involves engaging in cognitions and behaviours to change the environment and thus reduce the impact of the stressful situation. Emotion-focused coping involves dealing with the emotional consequences of the stressful situation by either changing the way one attends to the stressful environment or altering the meaning of what is happening to mitigate the stress (Lazarus, 1993). The measurement of coping using the WOC scale enshrined this distinction, and because of its domination of the coping literature in the 1980s, the distinction has been adopted by others in developing self-report coping instruments (Billings and Moos, 1984; Carver *et al.*, 1989; Parker and Endler, 1992).

The distinction is, however, not without its difficulties. It is not always easy to distinguish between emotion- and problem-focused coping and in many instances a cognition or behaviour may serve both functions, such as with seeking social support (Cohen 1987). It has been suggested that in order to determine what function the behaviour is serving one has to understand the context in which coping takes place (Folkman *et al.*, 1986). This is an obvious pitfall to the use of questionnaires that dichotomise these two functions and increases the difficulty of interpreting coping attempts when the context of coping is often left largely unspecified, e.g., coping with 'your illness'. The distinction between problem- and emotion-focused coping may be too simple and it is interesting to note that Lazarus himself recognises the possibility of other functions of coping (Carver *et al.* 1989; Lazarus, 1993).

Not all attempts to reproduce the distinction between emotion- and problem-focused coping have been successful. Endler and Parker (1990b) proposed a similar distinction between task-oriented coping and person-oriented coping (Endler and Parker, 1990b). Task-oriented coping mirrors problem-focused coping whereas person-oriented coping reflects emotion-focused coping. Again there is some difficulty with classifying all coping strategies into this two-category schema. As Parker *et al.* (1992) note, avoidance may involve person-oriented coping, as in seeking out others for a social diversion, or task-oriented coping, as in engaging in a substitute task to avoid the stressful situation (Parker and Endler, 1992).

A more general difficulty in coping measures is the place of social support. In some coping assessments seeking social support is seen as a coping strategy (Folkman and Lazarus, 1988). Social supports can be used for both emotional and problem-solving coping. Seeking information or analysing the practical difficulties of a problem with a friend may be considered problem-solving coping. Using others as comparisons or as an opportunity to express emotions may be viewed as emotion-focused coping. The social-support dimension serves to emphasise the difficulties of classifying behaviour easily into higher-order categories which consider the functions of coping. One way of resolving the dilemma with regard to social support is to view it as a resource for various coping behaviours (Endler and Parker, 1990a; Parker and Endler, 1992; Thoits, 1982). Although this may appear as a neat solution for social support, similar difficulties of capturing the meaning or intention of coping to the individual occur with other coping strategies.

COPING WITH RHEUMATOID ARTHRITIS

One of the issues with any assessment of coping in a chronic illness is the object to which the coping activity is directed. Arthritis researchers have adopted different frameworks for their assessments. Some have examined how individuals cope with a specific event while others have been somewhat more specific in that they have tailored their assessments to examine specific aspects of arthritis. A third approach has been to assess specific symptoms of arthritis such as pain. These different approaches are reviewed next.

General coping measures adapted for arthritis populations: the Ways of Coping scale as exemplar

A large number of self-report coping inventories have been developed over the past decade, most of which have potential applicability to arthritis (Folkman and Lazarus, 1988; Endler and Parker, 1990b; Billings and Moos, 1984; Carver *et al.*, 1989). These inventories have been designed to provide a formal assessment of coping responses to the stresses that the individual confronts. It has been argued that they all suffer from a range of methodological problems (Parker and Endler, 1992). Several have been applied to individuals with rheumatoid arthritis. Because the Ways of Coping scale (Folkman and Lazarus, 1980) – and the WOC-revised (Folkman and Lazarus, 1988) – has been either used directly or formed the basis of many of the studies on RA, we will use it as an exemplar of the more general self-report coping measures used in arthritis research.

In its present revised form, the Ways of Coping scale contains sixty-six questions which are grouped into eight scales that were empirically derived through factor analysis (Folkman and Lazarus, 1988; Lazarus, 1993; see Table 7.1). The internal-consistency reliability of the scales as developed on populations of college students and community-residing, middle-aged married couples (Folkman and Lazarus, 1988) ranges between 0.66 and 0.79. (It is important to note that it has not always been possible to identify the same factor structure when the WOC questionnaire has been applied to different populations (Endler and Parker, 1990b); this will be discussed with reference to RA populations below.) The instrument asks respondents to indicate to what extent

Table 7.1 Coping factors in original measures and as applied to rheumatoid arthritis

Authors	*Date*	*Measure*	*Factors/dimensions*	*Analyses*
Original measures				
Ways of Coping				
Folkman & Lazarus	1980	Ways of Coping checklist	Problem-focused coping Emotion-focused coping	Rationally derived
Folkman & Lazarus	1985	Ways of Coping	Problem-focused Wishful thinking Distancing Emphasising the positive Self-blame Tension reduction Self-isolation Mixed problem & emotion	Factor analysis & item deletion
Folkman & Lazarus	1988	Ways of Coping questionnaire	Confrontative coping Distancing Self-controlling Seeking social support Accepting responsibility Escape avoidance Planful problem-solving Positive reappraisal	Factor analysis
As applied to RA				
Felton & Revenson	1984	WOC amended 45 items	Six factors	Factor analysis
Pearlin & Schooler		10 items	Cognitive restructuring Emotional expression Wish-fulfilling fantasy Self-blame Information-seeking Threat-minimisation	

they used each of the sixty-six coping strategies in response to a particular stressful encounter, using a Likert-type response format. The measure is stressor-specific and does not assume that the approach adopted for this stressful encounter is generalisable to another. It assesses what the individual claims to have done to deal with the stress and makes no assumptions regarding their judgements as to the efficacy of the coping efforts made.

One attractive feature of the WOC scale for researchers in arthritis is that it is possible and in fact encouraged by the authors to add or drop coping items from the inventory, particularly context-specific problem-focused items (Folkman and Lazarus, 1988). This seemingly attractive notion, however, creates major problems of attempting to replicate the original factor structure of the scale and comparing findings on the instrument between studies. In many ways the use of a modified – if more appropriate – version of the WOC is equivalent to using a different measure; therefore, a need arises to perform an analysis of the factor structure of the new measure and to make comparisons of findings between studies with the caveat that the measure is somewhat different (Tennen and Herzberger, 1985).

Some indication as to how the WOC scale has been applied to studies of RA patients is presented in Table 7.1. It is clear that modifications in the measure lead to different factors being identified. In many ways this renders the distinction between general coping measures and those specifically designed to assess arthritis one of degree rather than kind. However, the factor structure of the WOC scale appears to be fairly consistent when examined with samples of individuals with chronic illness (Felton *et al.*, 1984; Dunkel-Schetter *et al.*, 1992; Revenson and Cameron, 1992), and somewhat different from the structure obtained with general population samples coping with a heterogeneous range of events (cf. Folkman *et al.*, 1987).

One of the earliest studies to use the WOC scale as a basis for examining coping in arthritis was that of Felton and her colleagues (Felton *et al.*, 1984; Felton and Revenson, 1984). The coping measure consisted of fifty-five items derived mainly from the original WOC scale with some additions from the work of Pearlin and Schooler (Pearlin and Schooler, 1978). Six coping scales were derived through factor analysis, several of which fit both problem- and emotion-focused modes. Two other studies have used the Ways of Coping scale with Felton *et al.*'s factor structure; and all three studies found the strategy of cognitive restructuring to be associated with better psychological well-being and the strategy of wishful thinking to be associated with poorer well-being (Felton *et al.*, 1984; Parker, McRae *et al.*, 1988; Manne and Zautra, 1989). In addition, information seeking was also associated with improved outcome in the Manne and Zautra (1989) study. More recently, Revenson and Cameron (1992) used the revised Ways of Coping scale with a rheumatic disease population of whom 75 per cent had RA, and obtained a similar factor structure. Thus, the WOC scale appears to be highly usable for studies of RA.

Long and Sangster (1993) argue that the effects of arthritis are pervasive and that studies which address the problems of coping with arthritis do not fully assess the effect of the disease on the patient's adjustment or quality of life (Long and Sangster, 1993). Using a modified version of the WOC scale, they assessed patients' coping with the most stressful event they had faced over the past month. Thus, the stressor was defined by the patient, and did not have to be related to the arthritis. Wishful thinking was associated with poorer adaptation, a similar finding to those studies using the WOC with 'arthritis' as the referent, cited above. No relationship was found in this study between the use of problem-solving strategies and adaptation. While this study makes an important theoretical point in that patients with RA face and cope with other life stressors that may, at times, outweigh the stressors of the illness, without knowing what the patient was coping with, this approach provides no more understanding of how context influences coping than do the others.

Illness-specific coping measures

One reason for the development of disease-specific measures is that the selection of items for general coping scales may not contain the relevant problem-focused strategies for coping with specific aspects of an illness. For example, samples on which the WOC was revised involved undergraduate students facing examinations and married couples facing a variety of minor and major life stressors (Folkman and Lazarus, 1985; Folkman *et al.*, 1987). It is questionable whether the items developed with these problems are applicable to the study of a chronic disease with specific symptoms. One advantage of disease-specific coping measures is that they are able to focus on known symptoms and the experience of illness in eliciting coping techniques. Thus, they may provide more targeted information for understanding coping processes and developing psychological interventions.

But even with disease-specific measures there is ambiguity as to *what* they are measuring. Some approaches focus on a particular symptom and assess coping only in relation to symptom, as we will describe a bit more later. In the case of RA the symptom most assessed is pain and a number of pain coping measures exist. This in itself is interesting given that the stress reported most often by RA patients appears to be fatigue.

Other disease-specific approaches adopt a broader frame, casting the coping inventory within the context of 'How do you cope with your arthritis or illness?' (Newman *et al.*, 1990; Manne and Zautra, 1992; Felton *et al.*, 1984). This approach ignores the diversity of symptoms and the wide impact of arthritis on physical, psychological and social domains. In addition, individuals may interpret the particular question as being directed towards one aspect of their illness while others may consider the object of the question differently (Zautra and Manne, 1992). In essence, by phrasing the object of coping in such a broad manner, the latitude given to individual respondents introduces much potential variability in the responses individuals provide. The alternative of focusing on specific symptoms clearly overcomes this problem but introduces other difficulties. By being more specific, an understanding of coping with the disease and all its ramifications is lost. The former approach has the advantage of enabling the individual to select what they feel are the dominant issues with which they have to deal. However, research with the area of arthritis using this approach has not specified what aspect(s) of illness the individual is bringing to mind when completing the coping measure, whereas research with cancer patients has (Dunkel-Schetter *et al.*, 1992). This information is vital to understanding coping within its context.

The London Coping with Rheumatoid Arthritis questionnaire exemplifies the disease-specific type of coping measure and was developed for use with RA patients (Newman, 1990; Newman and Revenson, 1993). The questionnaire contains thirty-six items and was constructed on the basis of open-ended interviews with RA patients, existing coping scales, particularly the WOC, and specific strategies suggested by health care staff. It was felt that by adopting this approach it would be possible to identify specific strategies that individuals use in relation to their RA. Patients are asked to indicate how often they adopt a particular approach to their arthritis, using a Likert-type format.

As such, the London Coping with Rheumatoid Arthritis resembles the more general coping scales adapted for arthritis, with the exception that its content was tailored for the population to be studied. However, in their use of this instrument, Newman *et al.* (1990) attempted to overcome a difficulty with the other structured assessments that organise responses to a questionnaire by specific coping strategies and then compare individuals on the use of each strategy. Such an approach ignores the overall pattern of coping strategies that individuals may use. By applying the statistical technique of cluster analysis to the coping data, an alternative approach was developed in which individuals were grouped on the basis of their overall *pattern* of coping strategies (Newman *et al.*, 1990). Thus, for example, individuals who used both cognitive restructuring and wishful thinking to cope with their arthritis could be distinguished from those who used cognitive restructuring but did not use wishful thinking. This cluster analytic approach has since been successfully applied by other researchers in studies of couples with rheumatic diseases (Revenson and Cameron, 1992) and patients with long-term RA (Smith and Wallston, 1993).

The data using the London Coping with Rheumatoid Arthritis questionnaire will be used to illustrate and illuminate this important approach to understanding coping processes (Newman *et al.*, 1990). Briefly, the study assessed 158 outpatients with RA; based on their responses to the coping questionnaire, the sample was clustered into four groups.

Group 3 tended to be the most open and active in the manner in which they attempted to deal with the stresses of arthritis. They did not use denial, wish fulfilment, distraction, prayer or religion. They did confront their disease, refused to reorganise their routines, engaged in physical activity and expressed their feelings. The largest group (Group 2) could be characterised as passive copers and did not strongly embrace or reject any of the coping strategies. Another group (Group 4) frequently used rest, diet, religion and prayer to cope with their arthritis. The remaining group (Group 1) used denial and avoided others when in pain, reorganised their routine in the face of the arthritis and looked to friends for support.

These four groups were not found to differ on demographic, clinical or laboratory measures and were defined solely by how they coped with arthritis. If it can be assumed that the groups experienced the same degree of stress as their disease measures were similar, then the data provide an opportunity to examine whether the different coping behaviours led to differences in the impact of the disease. Indeed, Group 3 was found to have significantly lower scores on measures of pain, stiffness and disability, as well as higher levels of psychological well-being. The findings suggest that the pattern of coping style adopted by groups of individuals has an impact on the reporting of symptoms, disability and psychological well-being.

Newman *et al.* (1990) also examined an alternative formulation which maintains that the coping strategies that people with RA use are primarily constrained by their level of disability (Newman *et al.*, 1990). This is a weaker hypothesis for the role of psychological variables, as it maintains that their influence is primarily upon psychological factors and does not influence disability directly. The results showed that the four groups with different patterns of coping still differed on both symptom perception and psychological well-being. This implies that coping strategies are important even when levels of disability are controlled, and that differing levels of disability cannot account for different levels of psychological well-being.

Problem-specific coping measures

While the disease-specific coping measures we have described may have more specificity than the general coping measures, they still encompass a large range of symptoms. When asked what they may have done to cope with their 'arthritis' individuals may emphasise one or a number of factors such as pain, stiffness, disability, social constraints, economic problems, future uncertainty and/or the unpredictability of flares. Each one or any combination of these may be at the forefront when an individual responds to any of the questions on a coping questionnaire. It is assumed that somehow patients are able to form a composite summary view of their arthritis and how they cope with it. It may be more appropriate, however, for the study of coping to focus on the specific stresses of arthritis (Zautra and Manne, 1992). The disadvantage of this latter approach is that it fails to capture the attempts to deal with the totality of arthritis.

Pain is the dominant symptom in rheumatoid arthritis and a number of pain-coping assessments have been developed. For research with RA patients, commonly used measures are the Coping Strategies Questionnaire (CSQ) (Rosenstiel and Keefe, 1983) and the Vanderbilt Pain Management Inventory (VPMI) (Brown and Nicassio, 1987); the latter has recently been expanded and renamed the Vanderbilt Multidimensional Pain Coping Inventory (VMPCI) (Smith and Wallston, 1993). In addition, Revenson (Newman and Revenson, 1993) developed an eleven-item measure adapted from the daily measure of Stone and Neale (1984) to assess coping with pain (Stone and Neale, 1984); the same eleven-item scale was also used for assessing how RA patients coped with their disability. The various dimensions covered in these questionnaires are shown in Table 7.2.

Studies using the CSQ have demonstrated that perceptions of control over the pain and the absence of catastrophising led to higher levels of psychological well-being and lower levels of disability (Beckham *et al.*, 1991). In a longitudinal study, Keefe *et al.* (1989) examined the catastrophising scale of the Coping Strategies Questionnaire in 233 RA patients. High scores on catastrophising at Time 1 were associated with poorer outcome on measures of disability and psychological well-being 6 months later. Moreover, patients tended to be consistent in their use of catastrophising over time (Keefe *et al.*, 1989).

The VPMI has its origins in research in chronic pain and was designed to assess cognitive and behavioural pain-coping strategies. Longitudinal research with this instrument has demonstrated that active coping strategies lead to more favourable outcomes and passive strategies to unfavourable outcomes; passive coping during periods of high pain may be particularly detrimental to psychological well-being (Brown and Nicassio, 1987; Brown, Nicassio, *et al.*, 1989).

METHODOLOGICAL ISSUES

Temporal issues in coping assessment

A number of temporal issues deserve consideration here. These issues arise regarding change in coping efforts and coping efficacy over time and the most appropriate times to assess those efforts.

Table 7.2 Dimensions used in coping with pain questionnaires

VPMI	*VMPCI*	*Revenson*	*Daily pain coping*
Active	Positive problem-solving	Positive reinterpretation	Direct action
Passive	Distraction	Distraction	Distraction
	Minimisation	Thought about solutions	Emotional support
	Use of religion	Gathered information	Redefinition
	Vent negative emotions	Took direct action	
	Self-blame	Emotional expression	Emotional expression
	Self-isolation	Sought professional help	
	Wishful thinking	Relaxation	Relaxation
	Catastrophising/disengagement	Sought spiritual comfort	Spiritual comfort

One question is whether there is any evidence that the coping strategies change over time. One way to assess this is to examine the relation between disease duration and coping. Parker, McRae, *et al.* (1988) divided their sample of eighty-four patients into four groups based on time since diagnosis and found no differences among those groups in their coping strategies profiles as measured by the WOC (Parker, McRae, *et al.*, 1988). In other studies, no relation between disease duration and intensity or type of coping efforts has been found (Felton *et al.*, 1984). In the study by Newman discussed earlier (Newman *et al.*, 1990), the time since diagnosis was significantly greater in one of the four groups. This group of patients was notable in that no particular coping strategy dominated their efforts to deal with the stresses created by RA; instead, they tended to use each of the coping strategies but only to a limited extent. Together, these findings suggest that as the disease progresses, individuals appear to use a wide range of coping strategies but that no particular strategy (or strategies) is utilised to an extreme. It may be that with time and experience individuals tend to fall into a more passive response to the problems RA creates, or that they become more flexible in their coping repertoire.

As these studies illustrate, this approach has relied primarily on cross-sectional data and not intra-individual assessment of change. One study that examined coping over a 6-month interval found moderate correlations for each coping strategy over time, ranging from 0.34 for the strategy of threat minimization to 0.70 for information-seeking (Revenson and Felton, 1989). Thus, the evidence indicates that people may rely on the same coping repertoires over time, despite the fact that aspects of the illness, e.g., disability, change. In fact, changes in disability over the 6-month interval were related to changes in the frequency with which only one strategy, wish-fulfilling fantasy, was used.

A second issue concerns whether the efficacy of coping changes over time. Efficacy is most often assessed by the relationship between coping and a particular outcome, for example, depression or disability. Given the different issues that RA patients deal with from the point of diagnosis on, it is interesting that the strategy of cognitive restructuring appears to be an effective coping strategy (i.e., it is related to lower depression) across a number of studies of patients with varying disease duration (e.g., Felton *et al.*, 1984; Newman and Revenson, 1993; Parker, McRae *et al.*

1988). Similarly, the strategy of wishful thinking is consistently linked to poorer psychological outcomes both soon after diagnosis and with established disease, suggesting that it is an ineffective outcome.

The fact that these strategies are similarly effective in the face of different illness-related problems may suggest that they have a more general efficacy regardless of the specific problems confronted. Alternatively they may reflect the cross-sectional design of many studies. It has been assumed that the coping style influences well-being. An alternative interpretation for these findings could be that active coping strategies and, in particular, cognitive restructuring may occur when the individual is feeling psychologically strong and able to actively engage in problem-solving. Wishful thinking and more passive strategies may be engaged in when individuals do not have the psychological resources to positively tackle their problems. However, the longitudinal data provided by Felton and Revenson (1984) suggest a bidirectional pattern of causation, that while coping efforts influence psychological well-being, psychological well-being also influences coping choices.

A third and somewhat different issue involves the timing of coping assessments. The time period over which individuals are being asked to report on their coping behaviour has varied considerably across studies. With situation-specific measures of coping, individuals are asked to recall a particular event within a specified time frame. This time frame can range from 'at this moment' to 'over the last week or month'.

An assumption in these retrospective accounts of specific stressful events is that the recall of these activities may not be accurate. There is some suggestive evidence that recall of this nature is subject to a number of influences which may systematically bias the responses. Affleck, Urrows, *et al.* (1992), in discussing coping with pain, suggest that current pain level may systematically bias the recall of coping strategies (Affleck *et al.*, 1992). Frequent sampling and controlling for current pain level may overcome the problem of inaccurate recall.

When individuals are asked how they cope more generally within a specific time period, it is assumed that they are able mentally to accumulate and summarise their coping behaviours to arrive at a representative or average idea of how they have generally coped. While no study has looked at how well individuals are able to perform this extremely complex cognitive task, it would seem likely that it would be subject to a range of influences, including the mood of the individual influencing their recall.

On the assumption that coping may change over time, a related issue in the assessment for chronic illness is the time interval that should be studied. This becomes particularly important when examining how an individual attempts to cope with a *chronic* stressor. If too long a time period is used, researchers may obtain only a sketchy summary of coping efforts. On the other hand, sampling too frequently may provide unnecessarily detailed information regarding the flux of coping on a day-to-day basis but fail to provide an overall perspective on how coping is related to adaptational outcomes. If one adopts a transactional approach to coping, it may be advisable to schedule assessments to capture the 'real' changes in illness and disability, e.g., beginning a new treatment plan, after joint-replacement surgery, before, during and after an illness flare; in essence this would require a conceptualisation of 'illness time' vs 'real time', but might make temporal comparisons among individuals difficult.

When coping has been assessed repeatedly over time, the frequency with which it may be assessed has varied. A large variety of sampling rates has occurred in studies of coping with pain. Keefe *et al.* sampled coping with pain over a 6-month period and found little variation in the use of the coping strategy of catastrophising ($r = 0.81$) (Keefe *et al.*, 1989). In contrast, Affleck, Urrows, *et al.* (1992) sampled coping with pain on a daily basis using the instrument developed by Stone & Neale (Stone and Neale, 1984). In order to obtain a representative picture of coping over a reasonable period of time they sampled behaviour over 75 days and cumulated the responses for coping, pain and well-being. This technique provides information on the range and number of coping strategies used over time. For example, the mean number of different coping strategies used over time was 4.7 (sd 2.0) and 10 per cent of patients used only one coping strategy. These individual differences in range and variety of coping efforts were found to be related to background factors such as gender and disability.

Flexibility of coping efforts

The ability to change one's coping behaviour in response to situational demands or feedback has been viewed by some researchers as leading to a more successful adaptation. This is contrasted with an approach in which the individual rigidly responds to the same stressor or to different stressors with the same coping responses. There is some laboratory-based evidence that the majority of individuals are flexible in their coping (Kohlman, 1993). Similar evidence exists within studies of RA patients. Newman *et al.* found that 66 per cent of their sample of RA patients were flexible in their attempts to cope with arthritis (Newman *et al.*, 1990), with most of these patients having disease of long duration. Similarly, Revenson and Felton found that RA patients used a variety of coping strategies to a moderate degree (Revenson and Felton, 1989). It may be that over time individuals with arthritis move into a more flexible approach to coping and that their responses are less dominated by a particular mode or modes of coping.

It seems logical that some degree of flexibility in dealing with the variety of stressors and contexts in coping with arthritis may be the most effective technique to maintain psychological well-being. Blalock *et al.* found that those arthritis patients who used a large number of coping strategies (no matter what the content of the strategy) had better psychological well-being than those who used fewer strategies (Blalock and DeVellis, 1992). Affleck, Urrows, *et al.* (1992), in their examination of daily pain coping, found that individuals who reported using the greatest number of distinct coping strategies tended to have improving mood over the 75-day period of study (Affleck, Urrows, *et al.*, 1992). In contrast, in the study by Newman *et al.* (1990) the group of patients who used the most strategies to a moderate extent were not found to have the best adaptation to their arthritis (Newman *et al.*, 1990). Felton *et al.* also found that a greater number of coping strategies was related to poorer adjustment, perhaps because patients in distress were trying all types of coping in a frantic effort to find one that would work.

FACTORS ASSOCIATED WITH COPING

A number of factors make comparisons across studies difficult to interpret. Some factors revolve around characteristics of the patients, such as sociodemographic variables or personality characteristics. Other factors involve aspects of the disease process, such as disease duration (discussed earlier), functional disability and level of disease severity, as well as aspects of the social environment. These factors may be determinants of coping efforts, i.e., they shape coping choices, or correlates of coping that suggest a particular profile, or both. In this next section, we briefly describe some of the factors associated with coping that have been studied in RA populations.

Sociodemographic factors

Gender

As we discussed in Chapter 2, RA is a disease that primarily affects women. Consequently, most psychosocial studies have examined the coping patterns of women (see Parker, McRae, *et al.*, 1988, for an exception). Therefore, one might argue that the findings are not generalisable to male RA patients. As we discussed earlier in Chapter 3, the experience of RA may be quite different for women and our instruments have yet to access these differences.

Gender differences have been reported in some studies of coping in healthy populations although any differences have tended to be small (Folkman *et al.*, 1987; Pearlin and Schooler, 1978). Three studies using the identical coping measure but with male or female samples of RA patients found the same pattern of coping-outcome relationships (Felton *et al.*, 1984; Parker, McRae, *et al.* 1988; Manne and Zautra, 1990). Research in other areas suggests, however, it is possible that female and male RA patients might differ in the types of stress appraisals they make or the types of coping strategies they use. For example, women tend to seek support from friends and family to a greater degree than do men (Shumaker and Hill, 1991). It is even more likely that female and male patients differ in the types of illness-related stressors that they find salient or the ways in which the illness intrudes upon social roles (Lanza and Revenson, 1994a), both of which affect coping behaviour. At this point, however, research aimed at understanding the influence of gender in coping processes is minimal.

Socioeconomic status

Economic factors have been shown to have an important influence on coping. Individuals with higher educational or occupational attainments have been found to have greater coping resources and to use more effective strategies (Pearlin and Schooler, 1978; Eckenrode, 1991). However, it has been difficult to untangle the influences of socioeconomic status and gender in these studies as well as in arthritis studies. In Parker, McRae, *et al.*'s (1988) study the subjects were primarily male but of low socioeconomic status (82 per cent unemployed). In contrast, the studies of Felton *et al.* (1984) and Manne and Zautra (1990) assessed primarily women of average income. Thus it is unclear whether gender or socioeconomic status, or their interaction, influenced coping processes.

Age

Age has been identified as an important influence on coping. Two hypotheses have been proposed. The developmental hypothesis maintains that there are inherent changes in the way individuals cope as they age. An alternative approach maintains that the issues that individuals have to deal with as they age change and that these changes lead to different patterns of coping.

Felton and Revenson (1987) examined the two hypotheses presented above with a sample of chronically ill adults of whom one-quarter had RA. Older patients were less likely to use the coping strategies of emotional expression or information seeking than were middle-aged patients. These coping strategies were related to age even when level of physical disability was statistically controlled. The authors suggest that the age differences in emotional expressivity may be related to age-related shifts in the types of stresses experienced, but that the age difference in information seeking may be more strongly linked to cohort phenomena.

Two other studies of RA patients suggest that age might influence coping behaviour. In their study of 158 women with RA, Newman *et al.* (1990) found that the group of patients who used many forms of coping to a moderate degree, indicating flexibility, were older than the other three groups identified by cluster analysis. Not surprisingly, this group also had the longest disease duration, leaving open the question of whether it is age *per se* or experience with illness-related demands that shapes coping. Revenson and Cameron found that the group of RA patients and their spouses who engaged in active problem-solving coping were younger than the three other groups in their sample, but that this group was also the most depressed and reported the greatest degree of other life stress (Revenson and Cameron, 1992). In both studies, the question of whether it is age *per se* or the influence of age on the experience of life and illness-related stresses that affects coping remains unanswered. These findings suggest that age may not directly influence coping, but may influence other mediating variables.

Personality

Even though one may argue that coping strategies *per se* cannot be seen as indicators of stable personality traits, as they vary over time and situation, it remains possible that certain personality dispositions may predispose patients towards the use of particular coping strategies. Carver *et al.* suggest that three questions need to be addressed in this area (Carver *et al.*, 1989): whether people use preferred coping strategies across a number of domains; whether coping preferences relate to personality dimensions; and whether these preferred strategies wield an influence on coping with specific events. In their study and development of the COPE questionnaire with undergraduate samples, they found only modest correlations between coping dispositions and traditional personality dimensions on the one hand and coping dispositions and specific *situational* coping efforts on the other. From their findings, Carver *et al.* conclude that traditional personality dimensions may not play any role in situational coping.

However, personality characteristics may influence the manner in which stressful situations are appraised and therefore tackled. Scheier *et al.* (1986) suggest that individuals who are more optimistic tend to have a direct approach to problems and will not engage in avoidant coping strategies. Friedman *et al.* (1992), in a study of cancer patients, found dispositional optimism to be positively associated with active coping and pessimism to be associated with avoidant coping. A similar pattern of findings has been obtained among HIV patients.

The relationship between personality and coping preferences, however, has not been well researched in RA. Long and Sangster (1993) examined the relationship between optimism and pessimism among OA and RA patients. They found significant associations between optimism and problem-solving coping, and pessimism and wishful thinking. This study raises the question of whether these personality dispositions are predictive of psychological adaptation and whether coping behaviour is necessary to account for differences in adaptation. Optimism was predictive of better adjustment and pessimism of poorer adjustment among the RA patients. The use of problem-solving coping was *not* found to act as a mediator between optimism and adaptation, although wishful thinking mediated the relationship between pessimism and adaptation to some degree. One may speculate that these findings imply that many of the determinants of positive adaptation to RA may be accounted for by generalised personality dispositions and not specific coping strategies; however, the evidence is not strong. It is important to note that this study was cross-sectional in design, and as authors acknowledge, the mediating effect of wishful thinking may be accounted for by other factors.

Disease characteristics

Zautra and Manne (1992) argue that it is important to include detailed assessments of disease measures in studies of coping as these supposedly objective measurements may act as important determinants of coping strategies. From the studies that have included measures of disease severity or progression, it is clear that these are important to gain some understanding of individual differences in coping (Newman *et al.*, 1990). However, it is difficult to assume that behavioural measures of disease status, such as a timed walking test, or self-reported measures of disability, such as the AIMS or HAQ, remain uncontaminated by coping appraisals or psychological mood. The difficulties with the more 'objective' measures of disease, such as x-rays, that are supposedly uncontaminated by psychological factors, is that they have shown little relationship to other 'outcome' factors such as disability (Bijlsma *et al.*, 1991). As a consequence, concepts such as coping most likely mediate between disease processes and outcome assessments of disability and psychological well-being (Newman and Revenson, 1993).

The social environment

It is a truism to say that the social context wields a strong influence on how individuals cope with stress. The immediate social environment in which individuals find themselves, particularly friends and family, has been studied within RA and will be dealt with extensively in the following chapter. However, it is important to discuss here what effects the primary partner has on patients' coping efforts as the elicitation of social support is seen as an important coping strategy.

Manne and Zautra (1989) examined the impact of husbands' criticisms on their wives' coping and found a direct relationship between spouses' critical comments and wives' coping and adaptation to their RA. Patients with critical spouses tended to engage in more wishful thinking which led to a poorer psychological outcome. The authors argue that spouses' criticisms 'may encourage ineffective and even harmful coping strategies'. Patients who perceived their spouses as supportive engaged more in cognitive restructuring and information seeking, strategies which proved to be more adaptive to dealing with the stresses of arthritis. However, the husbands' psychological well-being was not influenced by their wives' coping or level of psychological adjustment (Manne and Zautra, 1990).

Revenson and Cameron (1992) used the WOC-revised to assess how individuals and their spouses coped with RA. They used cluster analysis to identify *couples'* (vs individuals') patterns of coping. In two clusters, the partners used similar coping strategies and were termed as congruent copers. One of these groups used instrumental techniques and the other did not have any strategy that dominated (labelled 'minimalist copers'). In one of the two incongruent groups the patients used cognitive strategies and their partners used few coping strategies of any kind, whereas in the other group the spouses used more emotion-focused strategies. Spouses in the two congruent coping clusters reported the greatest degree of caregiver burden. Moreover, the couples who used the coping strategies of problem solving, rational thinking and seeking support (instrumental techniques) were found to be more depressed and spouses in this group reported great intrusion in their lives by the illness and great life events stress. These data point to the fact that the illness affects both marital partners and that one partner's coping efforts may both influence the other partner's and affect psychological adjustment.

This study and that of Manne and Zautra raise a series of interesting questions, some of which a longitudinal study may well be able to address (Manne and Zautra, 1990). These issues include the question of whether coping strategies become congruent over time, whether when couples engage in complementary approaches to coping they adapt better to RA. In addition there is much research that needs to be performed to examine the particular influence that couples have on each others' coping efforts in order to understand how coping evolves, how the partners' coping efforts may influence adaptation, and how satisfaction with the relationship influences both coping strategies and adaptation. RA is a particularly interesting illness to study when considering these issues as it tends to involve female patients and male spouses, unlike many other chronic illnesses such as stroke or cardiac disease.

At a more general level, cultural differences in coping with RA have not been addressed directly. It is often assumed that information on coping with RA obtained in one cultural context is generalisable to other cultures. This acultural approach is not restricted to the study of coping but to many areas of the psychosocial context of illness (Landrine and Klonoff, 1992). At the level of more general health cognitions within RA there is evidence that patients' perceptions of controllability of their illness differ markedly between the USA and UK (Newman and Durrance, 1994). In order to obtain a better understanding of coping with RA it will become increasingly important to place any examination of coping within a more general framework of health cognitions which in turn are recognised to be shaped by the particular cultural context of the study.

SUMMARY

A number of methodological issues in the study of coping limit the ability to draw detailed general conclusions (Zautra and Manne 1992). Different definitions of coping, differences in the specification of the tasks and objectives of coping, inconsistencies in the definition of the dimensions of coping are some of the issues that limit a detailed overview of the advances made in our understanding of coping with RA. At a general level, research on coping with RA has produced some findings of improved psychological well-being with active problem-solving coping and poorer outcomes with passive and wish-fulfilling coping. In addition comparisons with those in a worse state lead to a sense of psychological well-being.

At one level these studies have produced interesting and important findings demonstrating that coping with RA or its symptoms has a significant influence on the individual's ability to adapt. Studies have made some progress in accounting for the variation in adaptation to disease that patients demonstrate. However, our understanding is still limited. In particular one may question how much our understanding of the adaptation of individuals to RA has advanced if our conclusions are limited to the level of generality of the findings described above.

A number of possible explanations may be advanced. Perhaps the most important is that to expect studies of coping to be able to demonstrate more than these general conclusions may be unrealistic. To expect a limited assessment of coping at one or two points in time to be able to predict psychological well-being or disability in patients is to overestimate the strength of the concept and the relative importance of RA in individuals' lives. RA occurs in the midst of many other complex life pressures and to expect an assessment of coping with RA to be able to account for much of the variation of psychological well-being ascribes too much weight both to coping and to the disease. The complexity of the task of attempting to understand the process of coping within general life developments, attitudes and cognitions to health care, the influence of relationships amongst others is an enormous task and it will require carefully designed longitudinal studies to advance the study of coping with RA beyond the general conclusions that have been achieved.

Chapter 8

Social support and family relationships

INTRODUCTION

A chronic illness such as RA magnifies the stresses of everyday life and creates new stresses for all family members. This increased stress may increase patients' need for social support, but may also affect those most able to provide support – the family.

For the past two decades the psychological construct of *social support* has been viewed as an important moderator of the relationship between stress and illness. Large-scale epidemiological studies have demonstrated that having close, meaningful social relationships promotes psychological well-being and protects people from declines in health, particularly at times when they are facing stressful life circumstances (Cohen, 1988).

A number of studies have demonstrated the benefits of social support for people coping with chronic illnesses, including rheumatoid arthritis. Again, the research reached the conclusion that greater support is associated with psychological adjustment to the illness, adherence to treatment, immunological functioning, and mental health (DiMatteo and Hays, 1981; Kaplan and Toshima, 1990; Kennedy *et al.*, 1991; Wallston *et al.*, 1983; Wortman and Conway, 1985). These findings have led to psychological and sociological research asking the following more fundamental questions, 'What is it about social relationships that is supportive? When, for whom, and under what conditions does support have its greatest health benefits? And when are the family's attempts to be supportive considered to be *un*helpful?'

This chapter addresses these questions for families coping with rheumatoid arthritis. Social support is conceptualised as a dyadic interaction between a provider and recipient. The chapter begins by reviewing the literature demonstrating a link between social support and adjustment to RA for patients and their spouses, and then turns to an examination of how RA affects family members' ability to provide support. The chapter concludes with a discussion of the applications of current research findings to psychosocial intervention and raises key issues for future research.

DIMENSIONS OF SOCIAL SUPPORT

In its broadest sense social support refers to a range of interpersonal exchanges that provide an individual with information, emotional reassurance, material assistance, and a sense of self-esteem. Social support has been defined in many ways. It taps one or more of the following components: composition of the social network, types or functions of support, and satisfaction with support. Definitions distinguish received or enacted (actual) support from available support (Barrera, 1986; Dunkel-Schetter and Bennett, 1990). Some researchers define support as a stable characteristic which differs between individuals, while others view it as a behavioural response to a particular stressor. Some locate it within the larger social structure (e.g., social isolation or social integration) while others conceptualise it as a more proximal social resource or aspect of the family environment. There is a considerable overlap among definitions; for example, many researchers use a tripartite categorisation of emotional, informational and instrumental support. However, the nuances of different definitions may provide clues as to how support works.

There have been consistent criticisms that the construct is too broad or vaguely defined to be useful in theory development or applications to practice (e.g., Barrera, 1986; Schwarzer and Leppin, 1989). A broad conceptualisation of social support is adopted in this chapter as it permits examination of a number of aspects of social and family relationships that are important to arthritis patients' well-being. Gottlieb's empirically derived definition is both broad and meaningful: 'Social support consists of: . . . verbal and/or nonverbal information or advice, tangible aid, or action that is proffered by social intimates or inferred by their presence and has beneficial emotional or behavioural effects on the recipient' (1983: 28).

Nonetheless, it is important to disentangle the structural aspects of social ties (a structural approach) from the types of resources that flow through existing social ties (as these resources are often referred to as the *functions* of support, this is known as the functional approach (Cohen, 1988; Kaplan and Toshima, 1990)). Social networks are the structural linkages among individuals or groups of individuals; the provision of support is only one function of these relationships (O'Reilly, 1988). Examples of structural measures are marital status, frequency of social activities, size of the social network and network density (i.e., how many network members know each other).

In contrast, the functional approach focuses on the exchange of social resources between members of the social network (Kaplan and Toshima, 1990; Wills, 1985). Functions of support most often assessed include: (1) expressing caring, love and empathy; (2) validating beliefs, emotions and actions; (3) encouraging communication of feelings; (4) providing information or advice; (5) providing material aid; (6) reminding the recipient that they are part of a meaningful social group and (7) social companionship. Often, this exchange of resources is perceived to be beneficial by the recipient (Revenson, 1993; Shumaker and Brownell, 1984), although it may not be associated empirically with health benefits.

SOURCES OF SUPPORT

In order for support transactions to occur, it is necessary to have a network of people willing and able to provide support. Social support can be provided by natural helping systems, such as family members and friends; through professional caregivers, such as medical professionals and mental-health workers; within social and community ties, such as clubs or religious organisations; and from groups especially organised to provide social support, such as support or mutual-help organisations.

Adopting a developmental framework, Antonucci (1985) conceptualised the social network as a 'convoy' of people who accompany individuals through life and provide needed emotional support and assistance, particularly during life transitions and times of stress. Members of the convoy include spouses, parents, children and close friends. Over the life-course, some members may leave the convoy and others may be added; however, very little change takes place in the core of the convoy. No one network member can fill all of an individual's support needs; instead, different individuals fill different support needs (Weiss, 1976). This conceptual framework also may be useful in understanding support processes over the course of a chronic illness, as support needs and providers may change over time. It is also important to recognise that the nature of families and communities is changing in response to wider social and economic transformation. Moral sentiments and political theories about who will do what for whom often bear little relationship to the social realities individuals have to negotiate.

SUPPORT NEEDS OVER THE COURSE OF RA

As stated earlier in this volume, the trajectory of RA is generally progressive, but the intensity of symptoms varies unpredictably. The early years of the illness are difficult for patients and their families because this is a time when they must come to terms with the abstract meaning of the illness for the patient's life and contend with a readjustment of the family's prior pattern of interaction. The more concrete tasks of coping with RA include adjusting to medical treatment demands, reduced functional abilities and subsequent changes in lifestyle. As the illness progresses, disability increases and flare-ups of pain and stiffness become more frequent. Persons with long-term RA may require increased support of all types: assistance with daily household tasks, information about treatment regimens and coping strategies, and reassurance that they are still valued and loved despite their physical disabilities.

Thus, at all stages of the illness, increased support may be essential for optimal adaptation. Family members may sense a need to provide types of support and reassurance that they have not been previously required to give. For example, many male spouses of RA patients have to perform household chores that were not part of their repertoire. This increased responsibility to provide support may lead to perceptions of burden, and health declines for family caregivers.

SOCIAL SUPPORT AND PATIENTS' ADJUSTMENT TO RA

Emotional support and instrumental assistance from family members may be the most important factor in patients' psychological adjustment to chronic illness and, consequently, the family's ability to cope effectively. Most individuals still turn to family members in times of crisis before seeking help and advice from professional helpers (Birkel and Reppucci, 1983). Any one family member cannot provide all types of support, however. Such expectations place a great burden on that individual, compromising his or her health. Instead, different people serve different supportive functions within the network, so that it is the support network as a whole which fulfils the individual's support needs (Weiss, 1976).

Beneficial effects of social support for RA patients

The psychological benefits of supportive relationships have been examined in several studies of arthritis patients. Compared to those reporting less support, arthritis patients receiving more support from friends and family exhibit greater self-esteem (Fitzpatrick *et al.*, 1988), psychological adjustment (Affleck *et al.*, 1988) and life satisfaction (Burckhardt, 1985; Smith *et al.*, 1991). They cope more effectively with the illness (Manne and Zautra, 1989) and are less depressed (Brown, Wallston and Nicassio, 1989; Fitzpatrick *et al.*, 1988; Fitzpatrick *et al.*, 1991; Goodenow *et al.*, 1990; Revenson *et al.*, 1991). The relationship between social support and better psychosocial adjustment appears to be robust across studies of arthritis populations with different illness durations, when extremely different measures of support are used, and in both cross-sectional and longitudinal analyses. Moreover, social support contributes to psychosocial adjustment after controlling for prior levels of adjustment, i.e., social support helps explain *changes* in psychosocial adjustment.

The mechanisms of support: three theoretical frameworks

Social support enables recipients to use effective coping strategies by helping them come to a better understanding of the problem faced, increasing motivation to take instrumental action, and reducing emotional stress, which may impede other coping efforts (Cohen, 1988; Thoits, 1986). In addition, support may encourage healthier actions, thus preventing or minimising illness and symptom reporting (Cohen, 1988; Wallston *et al.*, 1983). Social support may also be directly related to immune functioning (Kennedy *et al.*, 1991). A number of models have been developed to understand the mechanisms underlying the beneficial effects of social relationships.

The stress-buffering model

A major focus in the social support literature has been whether support is more beneficial for persons facing greater stress or whether its benefits are independent of stress level. These are termed the *stress-buffering* and *direct-effects* hypotheses, respectively (Cohen and Wills, 1985). The direct-effects hypothesis suggests that support is beneficial for all individuals, regardless of the presence of stress or the degree of stress experienced. For example, emotional support may lessen anxiety no matter how serious the illness is. In contrast, in the stress-buffering hypothesis, the beneficial effects of support are stronger for individuals facing high levels of illness-related stress. Here, emotional support would be most anxiety-relieving when the patient is in a great deal of pain or about to undergo a major medical treatment. According to the stress-buffering hypothesis, social support yields its greatest benefits during times of stress, by enhancing the individual's coping efforts (see also Thoits, 1986).

The direct-effects and stress-buffering hypotheses have been compared most often in research using large samples of community-residing individuals who have experienced different degrees of stressful life circumstances (Berkman, 1985; Cohen and Wills, 1985; Kessler and McLeod, 1985). Overall, direct effects for support tend to emerge when support is conceptualised in structural terms, such as social integration. Stress-buffering effects are more often found when the functions of support or satisfaction with support are measured (Cohen and Wills, 1985).

A number of studies have compared the direct-effects and stress-buffering hypotheses among persons diagnosed with rheumatoid arthritis. Two studies found support for the direct-effects hypothesis only. Fitzpatrick *et al.* (1988) found that greater social support was associated with greater self-esteem and lower depression, regardless of the patient's degree of disability. Revenson *et al.* (1991), in a study of 101 recently diagnosed RA patients, found that the more support patients received, the less depression they experienced, regardless of their level of disease severity as rated by their physicians.

Two other studies present results that support both the direct-effects and stress-buffering hypotheses. Affleck *et al.* (1988) found reported psychosocial adjustment, as rated by a health professional, was lowest among RA patients with high functional disability who *also* reported dissatisfaction with the support they received. Brown, Wallston and Nicassio (1989) compared the direct-effects and stress-buffering models in a longitudinal study of 233 RA patients. High stress was operationalised as severe pain, and psychological adjustment was measured by a standard depression scale, the Beck Depression Inventory. In cross-sectional analyses (i.e., when social support and depression were measured at the same time), strong evidence for the direct-effects model was found: greater support was related to lower depression for people at all levels of pain. Empirical evidence for the stress-buffering model was also found, however. Psychological depression was greatest among patients with high levels of pain who also reported low satisfaction with emotional support received from family and friends. Analyses predicting changes in depression across the two 6-month study intervals supported the direct-effects model, but not the stress-buffering model.

It appears, then, that social support may operate in multiple ways to enhance adjustment to the illness and maintain health. Social support appears to be beneficial for individuals coping with different amounts and types of arthritis-related stress. At the same time, the greatest benefits of having social support may occur when individuals are coping with a great deal of stress that taxes their coping resources.

Social support may prevent the occurrence of additional illness-related stressors, or minimise the impact of recurrent ones over time. Gore (1981: 203) has referred to this as the 'preventive support function'. Social support from others reinforces the use of more effective coping strategies, increases feelings of self-efficacy and self-worth, provides motivation to take action, and reduces emotional distress that may impede other coping efforts or create additional stresses. Although none of the arthritis studies cited above directly tests this, evidence for this prevention function has been found in a study of community-living elderly (Russell and Cutrona, 1991).

The matching hypothesis

Another theoretical perspective suggests that social support is most beneficial when it matches the characteristics of the stressor faced. The *matching hypothesis* (Cohen, 1988; Cutrona and Russell, 1990) maintains that certain types of social support are beneficial when they fit the contextual features of the stressor. These features include the desirability, controllability, duration and timing of the stressor, as well as intrusion into social roles.

As has been emphasised throughout this volume, RA involves multiple stressors, including pain, declines in functional ability, flares, a demanding treatment regimen, somatic 'side effects' of medication, and coming to terms with the uncertainty and chronicity of the condition. Not every patient experiences all of the stressors, or all of these stressors at once. It is quite possible that social support may have different effects for different illness-related stressors at different times in the course of the illness. For example, support received by patients with severe and permanent disability may have negative consequences because it highlights the patient's inability to reciprocate that support in the present or the future (Revenson *et al.*, 1983). If people feel they will not be able to return the support, they may be less likely to seek help or to accept it when offered; they also are more likely to feel that accepting help will diminish their self-worth and autonomy. In Goodenow *et al.*'s (1990) study of women with RA, equity in relationships was strongly associated with greater satisfaction with support and lower levels of psychological depression.

The matching hypothesis also suggests that the effectiveness of support may hinge on a fit between a recipient's support needs and the amount or type of support received. For example, a recently diagnosed patient may desire concrete information to make a medical decision, whereas a more disabled patient may prefer help with activities in daily living combined with companionship. Alternately, misfit may involve discrepancies between the amount of support desired and the amount received; if the support provided exceeds the support required, feelings of dependency may ensue.

The timing of support may also create a lack of fit (Jacobson, 1986; Revenson, 1993; Revenson *et al.*, 1983). The same supportive action may be evaluated as supportive by the recipient if provided at the right time and as non-supportive if provided at the wrong time. For example, Dunkel-Schetter (1984) found that emotional support was most appreciated at the time of a cancer diagnosis, when the major coping task was dealing with the emotions surrounding the meaning of the illness for one's life.

When is support considered to be helpful and appropriate by people with arthritis? Affleck *et al.* (1988) asked RA patients what people said or did recently that helped them cope with their illness and what added further strain to their coping efforts. The most commonly reported helpful gestures were: (1) being given the opportunity to express feelings and concerns, (2) receiving encouragement, hope and optimism, and (3) receiving advice and information when it was desired.

The matching hypothesis may be conceptualised not only in terms of the fit between support needs and type of support provided, but in terms of *who* is providing the support. Two studies of rheumatic disease patients examined the most helpful and unhelpful support patients received in the context of who had provided the support (Lanza *et al.*, 1995). In both studies, emotional support from the spouse and problem-focused (tangible) support from medical professionals (i.e., prescribing effective drugs and treatments) were perceived by patients as most helpful. Mirroring this finding, a lack of emotional support from spouses and ineffective problem-focused support from medical professionals were seen as most *un*helpful. Unwanted or unsolicited advice from close friends was also perceived as unhelpful, particularly among recently diagnosed patients. These findings suggest that support providers often offer support to RA patients that does not match the patients' needs. One patient in a study by Revenson *et al.* (1991), whose depression was quite severe, stated, 'There are a lot of people around to support me. But they don't *listen*. At least I would do that for them.'

Social support as coping assistance

The transactional stress and coping paradigm described in detail in Chapter 7 (Lazarus and Folkman, 1984) treats support as a coping resource with the potential to operate in a number of ways. People must seek support in order to derive its benefits. Thoits (1986) reconceptualises social support as coping assistance; that is, support is the actions of others to assist an individual in his or her coping efforts. Thoits focuses on the similarities of coping functions as expressed by Lazarus and Folkman (1984), and social support functions (e.g., Cohen, 1988). For example, both problem-focused coping and instrumental support are aimed directly at solving or managing the stressor. Emotion-focused coping and emotional support are directed at reducing the distress engendered by the illness. Thus, the assistance provided by others through supportive actions should match the individual's coping goals, again suggesting a matching hypothesis.

Social support intercedes at a number of points in the coping process. It is an important element in the individual's appraisal of situations as stressful ones requiring active coping efforts. Information from others may influence the mental representations of an illness-related stressor and its seriousness for future functioning. For example, family members may be able to help a recently diagnosed RA patient put the illness into perspective. Social comparisons with similar others may also be useful in shaping stress appraisals (Affleck *et al.,* 1987; Blalock *et al.*, 1989).

Seeking support is a frequently reported behavioural coping strategy. By seeking support, individuals can obtain support that fulfils the major functions: patients can share emotional concerns with others (emotional support), request specific resources or assistance (instrumental or tangible support), or obtain feedback about their coping choices (informational support). Through these transactions, individuals may feel more secure in their coping abilities (self-efficacy) and gain a greater sense of self-worth and competence (esteem support). Support may also help patients maintain their coping efforts. Positive feedback from valued others may bolster damaged self-esteem, foster a sense of optimism, or reinforce successful coping efforts. Informational support may provide new coping solutions. Simply feeling that others are being supportive may increase the likelihood that positive coping behaviours will be continued.

The costs of receiving support

Most of the social support literature has focused on its benefits for individual and family well-being. Yet receiving, using or requesting social support have their costs as well as their benefits (Coyne *et al.,* 1988; Revenson, 1993; Revenson *et al.,* 1991). In order to maximise the benefits and minimise the costs of family support, it is important to understand how support can both help *and* hinder adjustment to rheumatic disease.

Evidence that supportive relationships sometimes act more as a 'stressor' than a 'stress-buffer' has been found among other medical populations, including cancer patients (Dunkel-Schetter and Wortman, 1982; Revenson *et al.*, 1983) and stroke patients (Schulz and Tompkins, 1990; Thompson and Sobolew-Shubin, 1993). These studies suggest that positive and negative social interactions have differential and independent effects on mental health.

A small but growing number of studies provides empirical evidence of the costs of social support for arthritis patients. In a sample of 101 recently diagnosed RA patients, Revenson *et al.* (1991) found that problematic support from friends and family (measured by items such as 'gave you information or made suggestions that you found unhelpful or upsetting', 'found it hard to understand the way you felt') was related to psychological depression, even though the patients may have been simultaneously receiving positive social support from the same people. RA patients who reported receiving little positive support *and* much problematic support from the same network members were at highest risk for depression. Similarly, in a study of 103 female RA patients and their husbands (Manne and Zautra, 1989), critical remarks made by the husband (e.g., statements that the husband disliked, disapproved of or resented an illness-related behaviour or characteristic of his wife) were related to maladaptive coping by the patient (e.g., engaging in wishful thinking), which in turn predicted poorer adjustment to the illness.

What characteristics of support make it *non*supportive in the eyes of the recipient? Common types of unhelpful support reported by rheumatoid arthritis patients are (1) minimising illness severity, (2) pessimistic comments, and (3) pity or overly solicitous attitudes (Affleck *et al.*, 1988). These types of social exchanges lead to decreased self-esteem, loss of autonomy and decreased psychological well-being. Perceptions of negative support may be linked to the timing of support; support may be beneficial only at times when the individual needs aid and is receptive to it (Cohen, 1988). And support needs change over the course of RA, in response to changing treatment regimen demands, disability, pain and symptoms. What may be useful one day may be perceived as unhelpful the next.

It is important to distinguish between negative social interactions and well-meaning social-support attempts that backfire. The former involves criticism ('You never handle your pain well') and angry outbursts ('*Your* arthritis is ruining *my* life!'); these negative exchanges were never meant to be supportive or helpful. In contrast, many well-intended attempts at helping go awry, for example, when relatives unqualified to give medical advice do so (Lanza *et al.*, 1995).

Another explanation for support attempts that backfire involves miscommunication between support provider and recipient. In a study of 35 long-time married RA patients and their spouses, Melamed and Brenner (1989) found that partners often disagreed about what constitutes supportive behaviour from the spouse without arthritis. Agreement between husbands and wives on which behaviours are considered supportive and nonsupportive was high only for a few actions ('expressed irritation', 'expressed anger', 'ignored me', and 'got me something to eat'). This suggests that communication between partners about expected support may not be adequate.

Supportive actions may also be interpreted as a form of social control. Although some research suggests that support from family members can increase patients' adherence to treatment, it may be seen as coercive behaviour, increasing rather than decreasing patients' resistance to recommended health practices (Rook, 1990). Medical practitioners should work with family members to encourage patients' coping efforts, provide emotional support and offer instrumental help that does not undermine the patient's self-esteem and autonomy.

It is important to distinguish problematic support exchanges from the *absence* of support, where no offers of help or statements of concern are made. The latter case may indicate social isolation, which has been shown to be detrimental to health (Berkman, 1985). The literature shows that the presence of support is preferable to the condition where support is absent, but it is less clear whether receiving problematic support is better than having no support at all. Negative interactions among family members may indicate deeper and potentially longer-lasting problems – problems which are exacerbated by illness-related stresses. Low levels of spousal support may actually be an indication of marital discord, and it is this discord, and not the lack of support, which may lead to psychological problems. In fact, problematic family relationships may be in themselves sources of stress (Coyne and DeLongis, 1986).

SPOUSES OF RA PATIENTS AS PROVIDERS AND RECIPIENTS OF SUPPORT

Spouses, in particular, bear a large proportion of the stresses and burdens engendered by the illness. The spouse is often the primary provider of social support in a married individual's life. There are also societal or normative expectations that the healthy spouse care for his or her ill partner.

Spouses occupy a dual and sometimes conflicting role in the process of coping with RA: they serve as the primary support provider to the RA patient, but, at the same time, need support for the illness-related stresses they experience. In addition, the provision of support itself may be conceptualised as a stressor for the spouse (Revenson, 1993).

Living with a spouse who has rheumatoid arthritis can affect the partner, and the marriage itself, in many ways. Some patients report that their arthritis brought their families closer together, others feel it pried the marriage apart, and some say it made no difference (e.g., Revenson and Majerovitz, 1990; Pritchard, 1989). The research evidence for a causal association of RA with divorce is mixed. Some studies have found that divorce is more prevalent among individuals with RA, whereas others find that the divorce rates of persons with RA do not differ from those in the general population. Moreover, there is little evidence to suggest that the illness precipitates divorce or that the lower rate of remarriage among RA patients is associated with disease course (Medsger and Robinson, 1972).

There is no dispute, however, that rheumatic disease creates stress for the healthy spouse and on the marriage. As described throughout this volume, patients with rheumatic disease face a complex set of illness-related demands and stressors, including severe and often unpredictable pain, intermittent yet increasing physical disability, uncertainty about disease progression, and frequent medical care. These stressors create demands for increased emotional support and tangible assistance from the spouse and other family members. For example, spouses may be forced to take on new or additional household responsibilities when the patient is physically limited. Given that rheumatoid arthritis is more prevalent among women, these responsibilities may be outside traditional gender roles.

For the most part, research on the psychological impact of illness on the spouse has dealt with conditions such as cancer and heart disease, which involve life-threat and hospitalisation, or mental-health disorders, such as depression (see review by Revenson, 1994). Only a few studies have focused on spouses of RA patients. Moreover, most studies have dealt with mental-health outcomes only (e.g., depression), and not explored the broader range of quality of life outcomes affected by the illness. Few studies have examined how the stresses of living with an ill person affect a spouse's ability to *provide* support to his ill partner (see Lane and Hobfoll, 1992; Revenson and Majerovitz, 1990, for exceptions).

Spouses of RA patients do not appear to manifest clinical levels of psychopathology. In two studies (Manne and Zautra, 1990; Revenson and Majerovitz, 1990), RA spouses' levels of depressive symptoms were comparable to those of community samples, and levels of stress were moderate and comparable to national norms. RA spouses also report levels of marital satisfaction comparable to other married samples. It should be noted that in these studies, most spouses were men, and men have lower reporting rates of depressive symptoms (DeVellis, 1993).

Despite the non-clinical levels of depressive symptoms, spouses of people with rheumatoid arthritis (called RA spouses here) experience a great deal of stress because of their partners' illnesses. Revenson and Majerovitz (1990) asked RA spouses to describe the stresses they had encountered in living with someone who has RA. Without prompting, two-thirds of the sample reported changes in the marriage since the onset of the illness. Some spouses reported that they had grown closer to the patient. A number of spouses spontaneously described changes in the amount of support they provided. Some reported they were providing more support than they had before illness onset; others said it was difficult to meet what they perceived as increased demands for support on the part of the patient. A number of spouses admitted that the patient had become more moody or depressed since illness onset. As a consequence, these spouses found it more difficult to provide support to their partners. In fact, two wives confided that they had lessened their own demands for support, for fear of increasing their ill husbands' distress.

Spouses of individuals with chronic illness often experience depression and anxiety, marital communication difficulties and problems at work (Revenson, 1994). In a study of 103 spouses of patients with rheumatic disease, in which 75 per cent had RA, spouses reported the greatest intrusion of the illness into their lives in the areas of social and leisure activities, family activities and sex (Lanza and Revenson, 1994). Many RA patients experience heightened levels of depression and anxiety (DeVellis, 1993), and patients' depression may be a contributing factor to their spouses' psychological well-being. In one study of RA spouses (Revenson and Majerovitz, 1990), if patients were more depressed, their spouses reported greater levels of stress, although there was no correlation between patients' or spouses' depression with marital satisfaction.

The spouse as support provider

Another consequence of patients' distress may be that family members are less able to be helpful or empathic to the ill person as the overt distress chips away at their own sense of well-being over time (Coyne *et al.*, 1990; Dunkel-Schetter and Wortman, 1982). The RA patients in Revenson and Majerovitz' study reported receiving less support from their husbands or wives, and reported greater marital conflict when their *spouses* were more depressed. In a study of patients with pulmonary disease and their supporters, Lane and Hobfoll (1992) found that patients' anger was somehow conveyed to their supporters, who responded over time to this anger with their own increased anger. Thus, patients' emotions may radiate to their spouses, which in turn affects spouses' ability to be effective support providers.

The fact that chronic illnesses such as RA require spouses to provide continual emotional and tangible support to patients coping with persistent pain, increasing disability, and an unpredictable illness course may also lessen a spouse's ability to be supportive. They simply may get worn down. In a study of primary caregivers to stroke patients, caregivers reported a two-fold increase in the negative aspects of providing support over a 6-month period (Schulz and Tompkins, 1990).

Social support for spouses of RA patients

Most research on coping with chronic illness has characterised the spouse as support *provider* within the marital relationship. However, spouses also need support for the illness-related stresses they experience. Where do spouses and other family members draw their support? This may be most salient for spouses, who, unlike many adult children, live with the ill person on a 24-hour-a-day basis. The partner with RA may be less able to provide support in a marriage when they are in great pain or feeling depressed. Moreover, as suggested by some comments made by RA spouses (Revenson and Majerovitz, 1990), spouses may be reluctant to add to the RA patient's distress by seeking support from them. In fact, spouses in that study reported confiding less in the patients than the patients reported confiding in them.

Only about one-third of the healthy spouses in the Revenson and Majerovitz study had sought professional help from mental-health professionals or had participated in a support group. Instead, statistical analyses indicated that support from naturally occurring social ties outside the marriage served as a valuable coping resource. The RA spouses who received support outside the marital relationship were able to be more supportive within the marriage (Revenson and Majerovitz, 1991).

Support received from close family and friends was particularly beneficial for spouses whose partners had severe disease, suggesting a stress-buffering mechanism. The highest depression scores were found among those spouses with few social resources outside the marriage whose partners had become more ill over the past year and a half. The fact that network support, rather than support from the husband or wife with RA, played this stress-buffering role suggests that social resources external to the marriage may be critical when couples face taxing illness demands. Support from other family members and friends may alleviate some of the burden of providing care; alternatively, they may provide a safe outlet for expressing negative emotions concerning the patient and the chronic strains that living with an ill spouse presents.

IMPLICATIONS FOR CLINICAL PRACTICE

One of the great appeals of social support is that it is amenable to change through psychosocial intervention. Recognising that family relationships can be liabilities as well as assets, and that RA affects the well-being of all members, several issues of concern to health-care professionals are discussed.

Social support involves a reciprocal relationship between provider and recipient. By focusing on the relationship, support interventions can be directed toward a number of goals: (1) teaching patients how to develop and maintain family ties; (2) teaching patients how to recognise and accept the help and emotional encouragement provided by family members; (3) improving family members' skills for sensing patients' support needs and offering help; and (4) facilitating positive appraisals of support. These four goals are not mutually exclusive. For example, interventions that help patients or family members more positively evaluate the meaning of the illness in their lives, or offer more helpful support to each other, might affect a more long-term goal of strengthening family ties.

Application of research to intervention

Most support interventions and patient education efforts have been designed with the patient as the target of the intervention (Daltroy, 1993; Lanza and Revenson, 1993). But as is evident from the research presented in this chapter, family relationships in themselves are a fruitful locus for intervention. The practitioner's overarching goal should to be help family members cope with their relative's illness while teaching them how to be more effective support providers.

The research described earlier in this chapter can be translated into intervention strategies and integrated into regular clinical practice. Many of the unplanned negative outcomes of social-support transactions result from miscommunication or misinterpretation of the need for support. Thus, basic interventions might strengthen communication skills among family members. By focusing on how the illness affects the marriage (rather than either individual), practitioners can help wives and husbands to understand each other's perspective. Discussions could involve how spouses feel about providing and receiving help from each other, and how to identify when the help offered might upset or anger the recipient. In Revenson and Majerovitz's (1990) study, for example, many of the RA spouses expressed concerns of burdening the patient with their own worries, and hesitated to ask the ill partner for support; yet the patients wanted to be able to maintain their role as 'caring spouse' despite their illness and disability.

Family members who serve as support providers may also need support themselves; thus, some intervention strategies might target the spouse as the locus of intervention. Building support networks outside the marriage, both within existing opportunities, such as neighbourhood and work environments, or through other avenues, such as organised support groups, may provide critical social resources to call upon in times of need. While these networks may become more critical for the spouse's well-being as the patient's health declines and disability increases, network-building should be encouraged in the early stages of the illness. In this way, extended networks are in place later on. This prevention strategy may be even more important for men, who make up the majority of spouses of people with rheumatic disease. For men, the marital partner is the primary (and sometimes sole) social tie, and men have fewer close ties and are less likely to seek support from them (Shumaker and Hill, 1991).

Spouses should be actively involved in ongoing patient education and rehabilitative treatment. Agras (1989) found that individuals with stronger support systems adhered better to treatment, and concluded that it would be wise to involve the spouse in treatment of rheumatic conditions. Daltroy and Godin (1989) found that spouses' self-reported approval of an exercise programme predicted cardiac patients' participation. These findings suggest extending the inclusion of spouses in rehabilitative and psychosocial interventions to general medical visits. Family members need to understand the nature and severity of the patient's illness and treatment in order to be helpful. Informing family members of such simple things as the up-and-down course of arthritis flares, and what to expect when flares occur, may serve to minimise distress and uncertainty. The emotions and feelings of family members about living with a chronically ill person can also be addressed during routine medical visits. Although the practitioner may feel responsible for the patient's physical health, the psychological well-being of family members directly and indirectly affects the patient's response to treatment.

The practitioner can also serve as an information source for community resources, such as support groups, psychological counselling available within the hospital, and patient education programmes. In the United States, the Arthritis Foundation sponsors structured self-help courses for patients in many cities and towns; family members are encouraged to attend. This information is best presented early on in the illness course. Early intervention can strengthen existing coping resources and social ties, which may need to be called upon later, and open lines of communication for family members. Although encouraging men to attend support groups and voice their fears may be more difficult (McGowan, 1988), preliminary research suggests specific benefits will accrue.

A few caveats are in order to prevent misguided support interventions. Although decreased social activities and greater miscommunication may be a result of chronic illnesses involving physical disabilities, most RA patients maintain healthy social relationships. This is achieved by altering expectations for support, learning to ask for support that is needed, ignoring bumbled helping attempts, and strengthening ties with people who *are* helpful (e.g., other patients with arthritis). Thus, all patients do not have a support deficit. Similarly, most patients who seek professional support or counselling view it as a complementary source of support, not as compensation for lack of support from their families.

TIMING OF THE SUPPORT INTERVENTION

Disease duration and stage are important aspects of the illness context, as they reflect specific treatment regimens and coping tasks (Newman and Revenson, 1993). Different types and amounts of support may be more helpful at different points in the illness, as the fit hypothesis would suggest. Skevington (1986) points out that early in the disease when diagnosis and prognosis are delayed there is a strong desire for information. In the early years after diagnosis, patients may be coping with minimal pharmacologic intervention and routine medical monitoring, requiring emotional and esteem support. If initial treatment recommendations are not effective in minimising inflammation and pain, then a more rigorous treatment may be initiated, requiring more frequent visits to the physician with more intrusion in patients' daily routines, noxious effects of the medication, and decisions to be made about treatment course. Over time, patients often have to cope with increasing physical limitations, requiring greater tangible assistance with chores of everyday living. At this time, patients experiencing a good deal of pain and disability might be extremely vulnerable to the effects of critical comments from support providers (Manne and Zautra, 1989).

The rate at which the disease progresses and the frequency at which treatment demands change are other factors to consider. A less rapid disease process probably allows a gradual and smoother adaptation, as anticipatory coping efforts may be made. A disease course marked with frequent transitions from health to illness, sometimes without warning, may prove a harder road to follow. The stress-buffering hypothesis suggests that support is most beneficial during periods when illness-related stress is high. Thus, support interventions that help patients cope with flares or joint-replacement surgery may be especially effective.

There is little research that addresses the issues of long-term support provision: how does chronic illness permanently change family relationships? How can long-term caregivers be effective helpers without burning out? How do patients feel about receiving more and more support as their disability increases? Most of the research findings in the social-support literature are correlational. Even excellent studies utilising prospective designs have tended to examine the influence of support at one time on psychological well-being at some later time. Thus, the presumed 'effects' of social support on adjustment may just as easily be the effects of patients' health status, psychological distress or social skills on the seeking, receipt and maintenance of supportive relationships.

Theories of support that conceptualise stress as a process suggest that social networks may undergo significant changes in the face of chronic strains such as illness (Pearlin, 1989). A number of studies of Alzheimer's patients have documented the burdens and health consequences of long-term caregiving (e.g., Brody, 1989). Research with cardiac patients and their spouses has documented the severe impact of living with a seriously ill family member for whom one is responsible (Coyne *et al.*, 1988).

The nature of rheumatoid arthritis – a chronic, long-term illness involving periods of severe joint pain, swelling and stiffness alternating with periods of relative comfort – affects family members' ability to be supportive. The social-support matching hypothesis suggests that support must accommodate to these changes. As social-support needs change, caregivers must learn when to give and when to withhold help, as providing too much support or providing it at the wrong time may produce negative outcomes, e.g., decreasing autonomy and self-worth. Research suggests that support attempts may backfire because individuals do not know how to provide long-term support or support that does not demean the recipient (Coyne *et al.*, 1988). This perspective echoes the view that social support is a dynamic interaction among people, and not simply a passive receipt of help. In one study, when RA patients became more depressed over the 18-month period, spouses reported greater stress themselves (Revenson and Majerovitz, 1990). This suggests that providing long-term support to a depressed, chronically ill person may become a psychological burden in itself.

Interactions with health-care providers change over the course of long-term illness, as patients move from crisis phases to more stable, long-term phases of medical care. For example, at the time of diagnosis, patients may require support from all sources, but informational support particularly from their physicians, as treatment decisions are made (Dunkel-Schetter, 1984). Soon after, emotional and problem-focused support from the spouse may be critical in adhering to a treatment regimen that must be woven into daily life. Later on, when the patient experiences a symptom flare, tangible assistance with daily chores may be important, and friends and family members may be able to provide the support.

Support groups

Our discussion of the effects of social support on patients' adjustment to illness has focused largely on support provided by friends and family members. Family members, however, may not be able to meet the patient's needs for a number of reasons. Family members may be under greater stress themselves, as a direct consequence of living with someone who has RA and is in constant pain, or because of the additional burdens of caregiving. Older individuals may have fewer close family members or long-time friends to draw on for support (Kane, 1986). Physical disability may limit social interaction and thus the maintenance of helping relationships. In these circumstances, the support provided by professional helping networks (psychologists, social workers, visiting nurses) or what is termed 'grafted support' (e.g., non-professional lay helping networks, support groups (Gottlieb, 1988) may be able to supplement or compensate for the absence of natural helping networks.

Mutual-help groups or professionally led support groups consisting of people facing a similar life stressor can provide a valuable source of support for people with RA and their families. Mutual-help groups, in particular, provide an opportunity for individuals with RA to meet with others in a non-professional, non-stigmatising setting, group discussions provide avenues for discussing problems and solutions, identifying ways to cope with long-term illness, and being reassured that 'you are not alone'. Other people who are coping well with their illness may serve as strong role models. An important aspect of mutual-help groups is that they provide an opportunity for participants to both receive and provide emotional and informational support. Research has shown that those involved in 'bidirectional support' have greater well-being than those who only provide or receive it (Maton, 1988). It is important to realise, however, that mutual-help groups may set up normative expectations which are more of a burden than a support (Williams, 1989).

Much of the research on support groups for people coping with chronic illness has involved broad patient education interventions with a support component; thus conclusions about the effectiveness of support are usually muddy. In one study that did isolate a 'pure' support intervention from a combined cognitive-behavioural-support intervention, both intervention groups fared better than the no-treatment control group immediately after intervention, but only the combined group demonstrated lasting effects (Bradley *et al.*, 1987). Moreover, the outcomes of interest in these studies have been medical indicators (e.g., reduced pain or disability), adherence to treatment, or knowledge. Within these domains, support groups have not been consistently effective (see reviews by Daltroy, 1993; Lanza and Revenson, 1993).

No studies of mutual-help groups for arthritis patients could be located, nor did any of the published studies consider network-building or marital communication as outcomes. However, research on participation in mutual-help groups among individuals with another musculoskeletal condition (scoliosis) suggests that there are emotional and social benefits to be derived from even short-term participation (Hinrichsen *et al.*, 1985).

Family support as an adjunct to professional treatment

Support from family members may serve to enhance lay or professional treatment interventions. This is best illustrated by an elegantly designed study by Radojevic *et al.* (1992). Patients were randomly assigned to one of three treatments – cognitive behavioural therapy with family support, cognitive behavioural therapy without family support, or education with family support – or to a no-treatment control group. In the behaviour therapy conditions, patients were taught cognitive coping techniques (e.g., visual imagery), relaxation and deep breathing. The behaviour therapy with family support condition taught family members how to reinforce behavioural techniques and coping. In the education with family support condition, videotaped information was presented to patients and their family members, and group leaders facilitated discussions but did not provide behavioural training.

The four groups did not differ in pain, depression, anxiety or physical functioning post-intervention or 2 months later. Although there was general improvement for all conditions across the study period, patients assigned to the two behaviour therapy conditions showed decreased severity and number of swollen joints (post-intervention and 2 months later) compared to the education with family support or control conditions. More importantly, immediately after treatment, the behaviour therapy with family support condition showed greater improvement than all other groups on disease status. Although the two behaviour therapy conditions did not differ at a 2-month follow-up, the behaviour therapy with family support condition maintained its initial treatment gains. The findings suggest that family support may be an important adjunct to behaviour therapy, although family participation did not produce significant clinical gains for the education condition.

RESEARCH DIRECTIONS

Despite a vast literature demonstrating a link between social networks and health outcomes, there is surprisingly little knowledge about *how*, *when* and *why* support works. This knowledge is critical to the development of therapeutic support interventions and policy applications. The chapter concludes by discussing three specific issues in social support that are particularly relevant for research progress in psychological adaptation to rheumatoid arthritis.

The importance of context

Too often, social support processes are studied outside of the context in which they occur. The seemingly simple question of 'Is support related to adjustment to illness?' must be qualified by modifiers such as 'Support from whom? To whom? Provided for what purpose?' and 'Adjustment defined as what? In the short-term or long-term?' A contextual framework for studying adaptation to illness, developed by Revenson (1990), suggests that social support processes be studied primarily within their naturally occurring settings or contexts and that the nature of the context will shape support-outcome linkages. Thus, contextual research can address the three theoretical frameworks described earlier in the chapter (stress-buffering, matching, and coping assistance), and provide answers to the questions of *when* particular types of support are effective for *what* types of patients facing *what* stresses at *what points* in the illness.

An early study of the effects of social support on psychosocial adaptation of cancer patients conducted by Revenson *et al.* (1983) provides a clear example of a contextual approach. If the authors had looked only at the zero-order correlations between social support and psychological adjustment, they would have found no relationship between degree of support received from family and friends and psychological outcomes (negative affect, self-esteem, mastery, personal growth, acceptance of the patient role). However, when the sample was disaggregated according to a meaningful contextual variable – whether the patient was currently undergoing chemotherapy treatments or not – the pattern of correlations between support and adjustment differed between the two 'contextually identified' groups. For patients undergoing chemotherapy, support was largely unrelated to adjustment. For patients *not* undergoing chemotherapy, the pattern of correlations indicated that greater receipt of support was associated with poorer adjustment outcomes. Thus, meaningful aspects of the stress context affected whether support was helpful or not.

Measurement of social support

Several recent reviews point to the need for greater conceptual clarity and measurement development if social support research is to progress (Barrera, 1986; Heitzmann and Kaplan, 1988; House and Kahn, 1985; O'Reilly, 1988). The number of existing measures reflects an appreciation for the complexity of the construct and the importance of using an appropriate assessment instrument. Clearly, no single measure can answer every research question.

The measurement of social support has been approached in too large a number of ways to detail here. Reviews and critiques can be found in a number of sources (Bruhn and Philips, 1984; House and Kahn, 1985; O'Reilly, 1988; Tardy, 1985). Instruments differ in whether they assess structural or functional aspects of support, received vs perceived availability, or satisfaction with support. It is critical to choose a measure of support that will be able to answer your questions of interest or test a specific theory. For example, different types of measures would be used to answer the questions of 'Who is providing support?', 'To what extent is support being provided?', and 'Is there a network of supporters available if help is needed?' (O'Reilly, 1988). A number of suggestions are provided for selecting measures which are able to examine the questions relevant to a contextual theory of support.

1. It is important to link support transactions to the stressors they are hypothesised to buffer (Eckenrode and Gore, 1981). Many measures assess only aggregated or global perceptions of available or received support, or satisfaction with the support received. The question then becomes, 'How specific does the measurement of support have to be?' For example, is it enough to measure support for your illness or does one have to assess support for coping with pain, disability, the treatment regimen, etc.? (The same issue was raised in the previous chapter with regard to the measurement of coping.) Although individuals differ in the illness-related stressors that are salient to them, too narrow a focus may limit the amount and types of support reported. One solution would be to ask patients which aspects of the illness are most stressful for them, and then tie measures of received support to those stressors (Dunkel-Schetter *et al.*, 1992; Revenson *et al.*, 1991).

2. Ideally, reports of received support should be tied to particular support providers (in contrast to a global assessment of support received from an unspecified network). Barrera (1986), among others, stresses the importance of identifying the specific source of support and understanding the nature of the relationship. In this way, one can determine if there are characteristics of support providers which shape the provision and effects of support. This

is particularly critical when studying chronic conditions, as the composition of the social network, even close ties, may change over the course of the illness. Thus, structural assessment of the support network is important, as it frames the support transaction, but is not a substitute for measures of functional support (i.e., the emotional, informational, tangible support received).

3. The number of social ties one has reflects the strength, quality or functional content of those ties (House and Kahn, 1985). However, the size of the social network and the social activities of ill or disabled individuals are often restricted because of the illness. Fitzpatrick and his colleagues (1988) found that RA patients did not differ from a community sample in the availability of and satisfaction with close emotional ties, but RA patients reported lower scores on the availability of social interactions with friends and neighbours. A study of physically disabled elders found larger social networks to be related to all forms of support (Morgan *et al.*, 1984). Thus, support measures should not be dependent on the size of the patient's social network.

4. If possible, the measure should assess multiple types or functions of social support. There are many categorisations of supportive actions. This will illuminate the stress-buffering, matching and support as coping assistance theories. For example, Wortman and Conway (1985) delineate six broad functions of support relevant to individuals experiencing chronic illness: expressing positive affect; validating beliefs, emotions and actions; encouraging communication of feelings; providing information or advice; providing material aid; and reminding the recipient that she is part of a meaningful social group (p. 289). These types of support may have differential effects on particular health outcomes or under particular stressful conditions. Similarly, effective support may depend on a match between type and provider or type and timing (Lanza *et al.*, 1994). The theory of support as coping assistance identifies specific functions of support tied to particular forms of individual-level coping (Thoits, 1986).

5. Given that support attempts can have unintended negative effects on psychological adjustment, assessment should include problematic or conflicted social interactions as well as supportive or helpful ones. The assumption that social support is a valuable, health-enhancing resource ignores the costs that may be associated with receiving, using or requesting social support. Negative social

exchanges should be distinguished from the absence of support, where no offers of help or statements of concern are made.

6. Measures of support may be confounded with the outcome measures they are predicting (Dohrenwend *et al.*, 1984). An individual's illness state (e.g., level of disability) may reflect a need for support, or colour perceptions of support satisfaction. Similarly, subjective perceptions of support may be influenced by the personality or emotional state of the individual and may not provide accurate information on how social support affects well-being (Heller *et al.*, 1986). Therefore, it is critical to be able to untangle the effects of support from those of affective state and disease processes.

7. The method of administration should take the illness into account. Physical impairments (e.g., deformities of the hand) may constrain some individuals' ability to complete either interviews or paper-and-pencil measures. Older individuals, or individuals with advanced disease or undergoing strenuous medical treatments may fatigue easily. Thus, the measure should have the flexibility to be administered in multiple formats.

Longitudinal research

Longitudinal research is needed to examine both the long-term effects of support on psychological adjustment to RA and the effects of long-term illness on social relationships within the family. Most social-support studies with RA populations have been cross-sectional, leaving unanswered the questions of whether support benefits can be maintained over the lifetime course of a chronic illness and/or what the consequences are of long-term support provision on support-providers' well-being. Stressors, coping efforts, and patterns of psychological adjustment are assumed to follow the ups and downs of the disease trajectory. Similarly, who is providing support at different stages may change over the course of the illness, as intimates become burned out during a long-term illness.

A few studies provide information on longer term support provision. Brown, Wallston and Nicassio (1989) examined the relationship of support to adjustment over a 12-month period for RA patients with assessments made every 6 months; path coefficients for a measure of emotional support indicated only a moderate degree of stability over the course of the study (the coefficient for Waves 1–2 was 0.57 and for Waves 2–3, 0.29). The stability coefficients for a number of measures of social support ranged from 0.63 to 0.80 in another 15-month study (Fitzpatrick *et al.*, 1991). In a study of hospitalised elderly, frequency of contact with network members (primarily family) declined over the first 8 months post-discharge (Johnson and Catalano, 1983). Elderly stroke patients in another study reported a continuous decline in network contacts over a year-long period (Schulz and Tompkins, 1990).

In a prospective study of recently diagnosed RA patients (Majerovitz and Revenson, 1992), the composition of the close social network, termed the convoy, did not change over an 18-month period for 70 per cent of the patients. Non-kin members were more likely to be removed from the convoy than kin, lending credence to the adage, 'Blood is thicker than water'. Relatives may remain more committed to providing support during long-term illness and may be more willing (or obligated) to weather unpleasant circumstances. At the same time, ill individuals may feel more comfortable asking for continuing support from family members, based on social norms of reciprocity.

More importantly, changes in the membership of the convoy signalled neither a loss of emotional support nor an increased risk of psychological depression. The overall level of social support provided by the convoy did decline over the 18-month period, but this decline in support was not associated with increased depression, even when initial levels of depressive symptoms and disease severity were controlled statistically. Why is this? During the early stages of a chronic illness, family and friends may rally around the individual. Once things have normalised, support may return to pre-illness levels. Alternately, the physical disabilities engendered by the illness may limit the person's social contacts over time and, thus, the degree of social interaction and opportunities for support provision.

Given that about half of the RA patients in this study who removed a convoy member replaced that individual with another person, it is possible that specific changes in network membership do not affect the overall fund of available support or satisfaction with the support received. The critical element to support's efficacy may be that needs are filled, even if different network members are providing the support. Patients with more severe illness were more likely to drop individuals from their convoy.

The day-to-day stresses of illness and increasing disability may have proved too much of a burden on weaker relationships. As Felton (1990) has suggested, illness taxes the individual's capacities and saps the individual's attention. Energies previously directed at social relationships may be turned toward other illness-related demands, such as treatment or pain management. Thus, shrinkage in network size should not be inferred to be a loss of support, but may reflect an active choice by individuals coping with stress to configure their social networks to maximise receipt of needed support without adding additional stress.

SUMMARY

The family is an important source of support for the patient with RA; at the same time, the illness creates stresses for family members that may affect their well-being or inhibit their ability to provide support to the patient. In designing support interventions, one cannot assume that difficulties in adjusting to chronic illness reflect a lack of support from the spouse, or that the patient should be the sole target of intervention. Clearly, the degree to which family members can meet each others' needs when one is afflicted with a rheumatic disease is an essential ingredient in both patient management and the family's adaptation to the illness.

Chapter 9

Psychological therapies

INTRODUCTION

Psychosocial therapies are increasingly used to treat chronic illness. First we begin by considering a number of issues which are salient to the provision of many types of therapy for patients with RA. Then we go on to present a synthesis of what is currently known about particular psychological therapies where they have been developed. While many of the interventions discussed here are directed at providing greater pain control or relieving depression, some have been designed with the purpose of helping people to live with their illness, while continuing to carry out their everyday lives. Throughout we have tried to indicate where new departures might be made in management and therapy.

THE COSTS OF TREATMENT

In economic terms the cost of arthritis to society is considerable. Major costs come from disability, co-morbidities, the medical services used to treat the condition, lost productivity through the inability to work, income support for the disabled and personal costs to sufferers and their families (Akehurst, 1992). Knowledge of these costs is likely to influence decisions about what treatment(s) should be used and for what length of time and this economic pressure will affect the development and more importantly the acceptance of psychological therapies in the same way that it affects decisions about medication and physiotherapy.

But the most important cost to the individual is from pain and suffering. There is scope for the development of new psychological treatments for pain and disability in this area for two reasons. First, there is evidence that existing medical methods are only partially effective. For example, in a survey of 180 patients with RA it was found that people who had undergone a surgical procedure and those who had taken drugs like aspirin or steroids were less likely to be working after one year than those who had not received these interventions (Yelin *et al.*, 1980). Second, effective treatment for the disease and the disability it brings will be needed by more and more people, as by most definitions, the prevalence of arthritis is increasing and the proportion of those with disability is rising too. This is especially true among the growing proportion of elderly people in the population (Yelin, 1992).

The treatment of disability must be a prime focus of psychological therapies for this disease, especially as psychological well-being is so closely linked to levels of functional disability (see Chapter 5). Satisfaction with one's physical disabilities rather than the lack of abilities *per se*, play a critical role in adjusting to RA (Blalock *et al.* 1993). Two recent advances aid the assessment of disability. The first is a new classification of global functional status by the American College of Rheumatology which takes account of the person's perceptions of their ability to perform self-care activities such as dressing, feeding and bathing, as well as vocational and avocational activities (Hochberg *et al.,* 1992). Implicit here is the assumption that these activities are desired by the patient; because of this, it is very much in line with current thinking about self-efficacy (see below). These activities are acknowledged to be age, sex and culture-specific. In contrast with earlier Steinbrocker categories, this new approach is based on patient self-report and is further advantaged by incorporating the full spectrum of activities appropriate to that patient which may or may not be fully appreciated by health professionals utilising the Steinbrocker system. The second advance is the development of a one-page self-assessment of disease activity, clinical status and joint pain or tenderness through the Rapid Assessment of Disease Activity in Rheumatology (RADAR). Results from this patient assessment show high concordance with scores from health professionals (Mason *et al.,* 1992). These two new self-report methods contrast with earlier instruments designed for physician use and underscore the importance of obtaining patient assessments of their own suffering.

SOME TREATMENT ISSUES

To set the scene for a discussion of psychological treatment and management, several issues deserve special attention. First in this section we consider some of the aims and objectives of therapy and then go on to look at the unstable nature of the disease, sources of fluctuation and unpredictability and how this affects evaluations of treatment. Lastly we briefly consider poor compliance with treatment, some evidence on the best times to intervene and the necessity of making treatment more 'social' in orientation.

The aims and objectives of therapy

There is still disagreement about what the objectives of RA treatment should be, but the principal medical aims are to reduce discomfort from pain and stiffness, to reduce disability and to restore functioning to more 'normal' or tolerable levels. Aims also include the minimisation of tissue damage, repairing tissue where damage cannot be prevented and balancing the good and counterproductive effects of medication. Psychological techniques, where they are currently used in rheumatology, tend to be viewed more as an addendum to the pharmacological armamentarium rather than as any substitute for them.

But what are the aims of therapy for the patients themselves? The reduction of pain is a primary goal for those seeking medical treatment (Young, 1992). People with RA want to be free from pain and to be able to carry out their usual activities; they are little concerned with their ESR level, the titre of Rheumatoid Factor or the activity of the joint scan. Yet the results of physical tests still tend to be given a higher priority in decision-making about treatment than what is known about the patient's subjective well-being (Deyo, 1990). Making a related point, Liang *et al.* (1982) say that while the objectives of therapy are to decrease swelling in the joints and improve their range of movement, these changes are not entirely sufficient to establish the success or failure of treatment. Health status measures like quality of life, happiness and employment need to be included to provide a comprehensive assessment. But what happens if a patient feels more satisfied and happier but still has uncontrollable synovitis destroying her joints? Is it then possible to conclude that she has been helped or not? While the use of multiple physiological, psychological and social outcome measures is vital to progress in this area it can also make interpretation complicated.

As pain and the loss of functional ability are so important, it is not surprising to find that treatment has tended to target these features, and the discussion which follows reflects these emphases. A contrasting view is that too much interest has been focused on joint inflammation and pain in the treatment of RA. Fitzgerald (1989) believes that a fuller understanding of the disease will require closer investigation of cardiovascular lesions or vasculitis, peripheral neuropathies and respiratory complaints associated with the disease. As such, complaints are bound up with the functioning of the sympathetic nervous system in arthritis. This offers scope not only for pharmacological treatments like the beta-blocker propanolol and the use of regional sympathetic block (see Chapter 5) but also for new psychological therapies directed at moods and emotions more than cognitions.

The instability of the disease

The fluctuating nature of RA presents a major problem in assessing whether treatment has been effective. Some patients recover spontaneously without any intervention as a result of the natural course of the disease. Improvement in pain following entry to treatment could be due to the specific effects of the treatment or to non-specific or placebo effects. However Whitney and von Korff (1992) have demonstrated that changes may be attributed to a regression towards the mean and this effect is most likely to occur when those evaluated in uncontrolled treatments are self-selected as a consequence of a flare-up. People in pain are more likely to seek treatment when it becomes intolerable but then improve regardless of the intervention performed. Those who seek treatment have higher levels of pain at the baseline than those who do not visit a doctor (Whitney and von Korff, 1992). As a result of using this heuristic, 'improvements' are more likely to be reported when in reality they do not exist (Tversky and Kahneman, 1974). It is therefore important to conduct more epidemiological studies where those with RA are not self-selected. Furthermore, those allocated to control conditions are apt to find alternative sources of relief during a long trial. While the randomised controlled trial is held to be the 'gold standard' for many purposes, it may not be the most appropriate methodology for studying RA because of its fluctuating nature (Lorig *et al.*, 1987) and more work needs to be done to reach a consensus about which alternative designs might be acceptable.

Rheumatoid arthritis is a widespread disease where a wide range of complementary and alternative therapies are commonly used (Cronan *et al.*, 1989, 1993). What is not known is how substances used in complementary medicine interact with the effects of prescribed treatment. Given the reliance of many alternative forms of treatment on the establishment of specific beliefs for their success, they could confound the findings of cognitive therapies which in many cases share the same aim. A few have direct and proven physiological effects like the application of soothing ointment using a rubbing motion which activates the gating mechanism in the spinal cord, so reducing pain (see Chapter 4). But more often the novelty effect of a new procedure or ostensible therapeutic substance has placebo power in relieving pain for short periods at least (Beecher, 1956). So any spontaneous remission of fluctuating symptoms following the ingestion of herbal remedies or using a copper bracelet, serve to spuriously enhance and positively reinforce beliefs that these unorthodox methods are effective (Pritchard, 1989).

Furthermore, mood fluctuations tend to accompany active inflammatory disease on a daily basis, so displaying the intricate interaction between physiological and psychological factors in the expression of this disease. In a prospective longitudinal study of seventy-four people with joint pain over seventy-five consecutive days, Affleck *et al.* (1994) found that the occurrence of an undesirable negative event during active inflammatory disease tended to be associated with pain that day, and in the day after the event. Those with no recent major life event had lower levels of pain, and those with a high level of social support had less mood disturbance in the day following an undesirable event.

Subsequent analyses of results from this sample showed how long-term reports of chronic pain and chronic mood in patients with classical or definite RA may be confounded with neuroticism (Affleck, Tennen *et al.*, 1992). Neuroticism is a characteristic of many chronic painful conditions and is not exclusive to RA as was once implied by those seeking evidence for a 'rheumatoid personality' (Gardiner, 1980). Although Crown *et al.* (1975) found that neuroticism was more likely to be a characteristic of those with sero-negative disease, possibly reflecting their anxiety about not having obtained a confirmed diagnosis, Affleck, Tennen *et al.* (1992) have not explored this idea in their data.

The unpredictability of the disease has been widely discussed in relation to this variability in RA (Wiener, 1975). While uncertainty is especially evident at the time of diagnosis and when the disease is mild, Affleck, Tennen *et al.* (1987) found that RA patients with intense pain often found it quite predictable. Those who found the pain most predictable tended to record fewer outlier days and briefer episodes of atypically severe pain. In cases where there was considerable fluctuation in pain and other symptoms, for instance where a relatively painful day was surrounded by comparatively painless ones, this begs the question about the accuracy of those measures which require patients to retrospectively estimate pain over a previous period and how this then affects their judgements about the success or failure of treatment.

Compliance with treatment

Motivating patients to comply with, or adhere to treatment for RA is a problem for most therapists whatever medium they use and however they define compliance. In this section we consider some of the factors responsible for poor compliance to treatment in this disease (see also Chapter 6). Three factors tend to predispose RA sufferers towards non-compliance. The first is lengthy treatment. The second is when the short-term positively reinforcing consequences from therapy may not be present (Achterberg-Lawlis, 1982). A reason which is commonly given for non-compliance is that if RA patients believe they will not benefit, then they are unlikely to carry out the prescribed action and this appears to be as true for performing exercise as for taking aspirin (Ferguson and Bole, 1979). However, in the absence of prospective longitudinal research this reason may turn out to be as much a justification for non-compliance as a cause of it.

The third is when treatment will probably result in unpleasant medication side-effects. For example physicians report a range of digestive disturbances from indigestion to major haemorrhage resulting from the regular use of aspirin and related compounds. The risk–benefits for available NSAIDs have been found to be less than ideal – ibuprofen is relatively safe but has limited effectiveness, indomethacine is very effective but has a high risk of side-effects (Downie, 1992; see also Chapter 2). While non-adherence to treatment tends to be viewed negatively by health professionals, there is a positive side which has not always been presented. In situations where drugs may pose a health risk and where the long-term benefits and side-effects of a drug have yet to be established, non-compliance may not be such a bad thing. A fashionable example is the long-term use of DMARD therapy in the treatment of RA where outcomes are unknown at present.

Other studies have used more 'objective' or indirect measures to monitor compliance. For example, a recording device attached to an exercise machine was used to monitor compliance with physiotherapy in a small-scale study of twelve RA patients (Waggoner and Le Lieuvre, 1981). Patients reported that a VDU helped them to keep an accurate account of their hand exercises. Often patients reported that if they realised they had forgotten to perform certain exercises, they would do additional work to return to the prescribed schedule, and this was borne out by the recordings. This study tends to support the view that non-compliance in RA at least, may be more the result of unintentional memory lapse than the explicit intention to cheat or manipulate, themes which are commonly found in this literature.

Reviewing nineteen studies of RA patients, Belcon *et al.* (1984) found that compliance with a course of medication varied from 16 per cent to 84 per cent. Compliance with physiotherapy was similarly spread, ranging from 39 per cent to 65 per cent, and adherence to splint usage from 25 per cent to 65 per cent. But the quality of these studies was poor, as compliance was rarely defined and only one had used a randomised control trial. Belcon *et al.* concluded that despite this lack of rigour, a reasonable estimate would be that 50 per cent or more of RA patients do not adhere to treatment, irrespective of the type of treatment they receive. Such findings raise important questions about the efficacy of therapy for RA as well as about the innovative strategies which need to be developed in this area to improve these compliance rates. Given that compliance with medication for the rheumatic diseases is not high, the search for alternative non-pharmacological methods of relieving distressing symptoms seems overdue.

Timing interventions

At what stage should interventions be performed? While most studies have focused on chronically ill and disabled RA patients with moderate or severe disease, more recently the focus has shifted to primary health care and such studies have provided much food for thought about where in the process interventions should ideally be placed (e.g., Lanza and Revenson, 1993). Mounting evidence indicates the desirability of an early active intervention which emphasises well behaviour rather than illness or sick-role behaviour. In studies by Linton *et al.* (1993), progress was charted for 198 patients seeking help for musculoskeletal pains in the back and neck. Some received an 'early activation' package which on average included one appointment with the doctor for a medical and a functional examination with advice, plus three sessions of physiotherapy. The outcome of this group was compared with those who had received the 'usual' treatment of 2 to 3 weeks of analgesics for severe and persistent pain and were conventionally instructed to 'let pain be your guide'. Those with a previous history of musculoskeletal pain reported greater satisfaction with the package compared with conventional medical treatment. But the best results were documented for first-time sufferers, who showed an improvement in activities, and had fewer days sick leave over the 12 months following the end of the trial. The risk of developing chronic pain was calculated to be eight times lower for the group who received the early activation package. These promising results pave the way for further investigations into primary health care – an area which has been sadly neglected in Britain.

One of the problems with treating painful chronic diseases is that it may be accompanied by depression, and the timing and type of intervention must necessarily take account of this. The incidence of pain and depression in RA is difficult to establish and has been discussed in Chapter 4 (see also DeVellis, 1993). Few studies have investigated the incidence of depression in non-patient samples with pain. It is therefore difficult to find out how far the hospitalisation process affects the incidence of depression – the business of becoming chronically ill – or whether pain alone predisposes people to become depressed. Indeed, results from some studies show that some pain patients are entirely free from depressive symptoms. Estimates seem to depend on the measures used.

hence the need for proper timing and intervention for compliance.

If depression is problematic for a sizable proportion of patients with RA, then this raises questions about whether the depression should be treated before, during or after the pain is relieved. Some of these issues require pharmacological answers which cannot be supplied here. But what can be tackled is whether in fact it constitutes a major 'problem' and one which those involved in the treatment of RA patients should be concerned about.

In a prospective longitudinal study of sixty-nine early synovitis patients newly admitted to outpatients, Skevington (1993) looked at whether it was possible to identify depressive cognitions which could point the way to a more fully blown depression. Before the first outpatient appointment, patients completed measures of depression, pain, self-esteem, beliefs about pain control and provided attributions about painful symptoms. This was repeated 10 and 22 months later, regardless of their health status at that time. Some had recovered, others were no better but had ceased to visit outpatients, still others had become inpatients or were awaiting hip-replacement surgery.

The results showed that depressive symptoms were at consistently low levels; at no stage in the study could the sample have been construed as clinically depressed and indeed there was a slight decrease in depressive symptoms during the study. Depression at the end of the study could not have been predicted by the attributions patients made about their pain at the time of admission, nor was there any evidence that experience of depression before the pain began primed people to depression once their pain started. There was however considerable evidence to show that both the pain itself and certain attributions about pain predicted how much depression RA patients reported at that time. At the time of admission, believing that the pain will be uncontrollable and that it will go on tend to be related to depression at that time, even though this is mild. Pain levels were particularly important 2 years after treatment began; degrees of affective and sensory pain predicted how much depression would also be reported. The belief that the pain will affect every area of life is also significantly associated with more depression at this time.

The clinical implications of these findings are that where pain and depression co-exist this is often not at all severe. In this study only five patients obtained scores which reflected severe depression, so the incidence of primary clinical depression is not at all common as some research would lead us to believe. However, it is clear that even subclinical levels of depression should be treated more seriously right from the start of treatment (Skevington, 1994). Also, the findings indicate that pain and depression should be treated together as a unit to provide relief from both, and treatment should focus on altering depressogenic attributions about pain. This could be done in pharmacological terms and by using re-attributional training (Forsterling, 1985). Recent modelling of the relationship between co-occurring pain and depression in RA patients with established classical or definite disease indicates that depression is more likely to have an effect on pain than vice versa (Parker *et al.*, 1992), although this may not necessarily pertain to those with early synovitis. Consequently, styles of cognitive therapy effective with depressed patients might be usefully applied here (Teasdale, 1983, 1985).

Making treatment more 'social'

Lastly, research on the treatment of patients with RA has tended to be largely patient-centred. Patients live in families and communities and research is sparse on how variations in this social milieu can influence the effectiveness of treatment (Skevington, 1995). 'Significant others' may have an important role to play in the reporting and experience of RA, as discussed at length in the previous chapter. Ward and Leigh (1993) found more functional disability among unmarried than married RA patients. This association was particularly evident at certain periods in the progress of the disease, for instance 5 to 7 years after onset, although it is not known why this patterning occurred. While the data support the view that marriage is beneficial for those with RA, this conclusion is controversial. An interesting study discussed earlier by Manne & Zautra (1989) has shown that spouses can inhibit or facilitate patients' adaptation to illness depending on the levels of hostility or support they show. Because the availability of good adaptation skills is crucial to the effectiveness of many psychological therapies this finding poses a cause for concern about whether the family situation is currently being adequately assessed. Many related questions also remain unanswered in this area such as what effect children in a family have on the adults' relationship and how this affects health status (Reisine, 1993). The influence of family dynamics needs to be more fully investigated to find out whether particular styles of interaction explain some of the variation in outcomes of psychological and other therapies in current use. Furthermore we may need to know much more about how RA families function as a unit before we are able to understand why some RA patients find psychological therapies more acceptable than others. Progress in treating RA will be hampered if research designs continue to use methods which assume that patients are socially sanitised individuals who can somehow be artificially detached from their social context.

COGNITIVE BEHAVIOUR THERAPIES

Behaviour therapy and its cognitive applications have been widely used to treat RA and other chronic painful disorders in the last 20 years (Fordyce, 1976). Techniques drawing on neo-behaviourist theory have been derived with the aim of controlling symptoms. At its most successful, such therapy provides a training in using techniques which may then be taken beyond the clinic to be integrated into a patient's lifestyle, thereby improving her quality of life. But more than this, such skills provide greater patient empowerment. Behavioural techniques have provided some freedom from the tyranny of drug-taking which is a daily necessity for many people with RA and an action which may last a lifetime if the disease is not self-limiting.

In this section we begin by considering the scope of cognitive behaviour therapy. Then we go on to look in depth at work on the main areas of psychological therapy. Readers are referred to a number of extensive reviews which have already documented many individual studies in this field and it is not the intention here to go over the same ground again. In addition to the overall picture, we particularly consider relaxation, imagery and social support.

The scope of cognitive behaviour therapy

The current scope of the components of cognitive behaviour therapies has been recently summarised by Parker *et al.* (1993) as including relaxation training, cognitive coping strategies, goal-setting with self-reinforcement, communications training, assertiveness training, problem-solving and training for the family of a pain sufferer. Typically, programmes contain the three components of education where a conceptual overview is provided, often with specific knowledge about the pain-gating mechanism. This is followed by a skills acquisition phase, where coping and optimistic attitudes are developed, and a final maintenance phase in which acquired self-management skills are generalised and consolidated outside the clinic. These three components are directed at improving a sense of self-mastery over pain. Several studies have shown that RA patients who perceive themselves as having more personal control over symptoms like pain (Skevington, 1983) and over the course of their disease see their illness as more predictable. Furthermore, this has a positive effect on their moods and other aspects of well-being (Affleck, Tennen *et al.*, 1987) and for this reason it provides the prelude to a discussion about cognitive behaviour therapy.

Looking at RA patients and those with chronic back pain and other unselected pains, Flor and Turk (1988) concluded that two sets of cognitions are central to the success of treatment in this field. The first is the patient's global attributions about her pain and her situation. The second is the specific statements patients make about their own ability to exert control over aversive sensations (see also self-efficacy below). Their results showed that between 32 per cent and 60 per cent of the variance in pain and disability in RA could be explained by these two types of pain-related statements. Cognitive therapy packages will therefore need to include and work directly on these features if success is to be ensured.

Relaxation

Relaxation has been used in cognitive therapy since the 1930s, but the term 'relaxation' covers a multitude of sins and progress has been hampered because the procedures used tend to be taken for granted and are therefore rarely detailed in reports. The most successful known forms tend to include elements of progressive muscle relaxation and training in the use of mental imagery. For instance, self-regulation techniques have been explored in the management of chronic arthritis pain for haemophiliacs. Promising results indicated that when practised twice daily for 3.5 to 5.5 weeks, progressive muscular relaxation, meditative deep-breathing exercises and training to generate images of warmth and warm colours gave substantial relief in terms of days without pain, and this persisted over long periods of up to 14 months (Varni, 1981).

Self-help strategies which patients use to control pain are affected by the fluctuations in illness. Affleck's group found that 40 per cent of patients in their study reported using on average at least one strategy per day over 75 days, like taking direct action to reduce pain or using relaxation to counteract it (Affleck, Urrows *et al.*, 1992). When neuroticism and pain-control perceptions were controlled in the analyses, it was found that those who used relaxation did have less daily pain. As relaxation is an integral component of many cognitive behaviour therapy packages, these results give support to its efficacy, especially long term.

However, relaxation has often been combined with other techniques in the search for symptom relief in RA. Pain and stress can be relieved by relaxation with biofeedback as an investigation by Achterberg *et al.* (1981) demonstrated. Significant improvements to pain, tension and sleep patterns followed training in these strategies or after physiotherapy, and this may have been because all participants learned how to relax. Here verbal relaxation with guided imagery and biofeedback about skin temperature was used to treat moderately ill RA patients who received two 30-minute sessions per week over 6 weeks. Improvements occurred in the biofeedback condition irrespective of whether they were instructed to increase or decrease their skin temperature. A related study confirmed that thermal biofeedback was superior to physiotherapy on a range of immunological and psychological outcome measures.

Studies on the role of stress in RA provide useful information about how the pain–tension cycle is intercepted by relaxation and biofeedback. Psychological stress was cited as a cause for symptom flare by 46 per cent of patients in one study (Affleck, Pfieffer *et al.*, 1987). Psycho-physiological studies of electromuscular activity show that compared to other chronically ill medical patients, those with RA tend to maintain higher levels of electromyograph (EMG) activity near their joints. Furthermore, during psychological stress, people with RA show greater EMG and electrodermal increases than those with other diseases and are slower to return to the baseline after stress. However, because EMG activity may itself be a symptom of RA and because there are methodological problems with these studies – particularly one of ecological validity – the causal relationship has not been fully established (Anderson *et al.*, 1985). Whatever the reason for these changes in activity, it is now much clearer why EMG biofeedback and progressive relaxation of muscles at affected joints provide some pain relief.

Imagery

The search for pain relief through psychological methods has also focused on the use of imagery. A range of techniques devised to manipulate imagery has been proposed by Turk *et al.* (1983). They claimed that the six main cognitive strategies they had identified like reinterpreting pain sensations and distraction, were equally effective in raising the pain threshold, improving pain tolerance, self-reports and physiological measures when compared to no-treatment controls. Considering a meta-analysis of the outcomes of fifty-one studies of these coping strategies totalling more than 2,000 participants, Fernandez & Turk (1989) found that over 85 per cent of studies showed that cognitive strategies have a positive effect on pain. Comparing the effect of each strategy with no-treatment controls and placebo or expectancy conditions, they found that strategies employing pleasant and neutral imagery were the most effective in relieving pain, while pain acknowledgement was least useful. They noted that in studies where positive expectancy conditions had been used, the results were no better than for no-treatment controls.

However, certain techniques have been shown to be more effective with particular diagnostic groups, as an early study of RA by Rybstein-Blinchik (1979) showed. Forty-four patients were allocated to one of four conditions which had been designed to assist pain control. Imaginative reinterpretation of the pain proved to be more satisfactory in reducing pain than either attention diversion or somatisation, where pain words were replaced by expressions like 'a certain feeling', or a control condition where the pain problem was discussed. The study did not, however, explore whether this strategy was used or useful outside the experimental situation.

Social support

How effective is cognitive behaviour therapy when compared to social support? Following random allocation of thirty-three patients to cognitive behaviour therapy, structured social support or a no-treatment group, Bradley *et al.* (1985) found that patients in the treatment groups reported a significant reduction in anxiety and depression at the end of treatment. But only those who received cognitive behaviour therapy reported less intense pain, showed less pain behaviour and had a lower titre of Rheumatoid Factor, implying that cognitive behaviour therapy may have a positive effect on the immune system. Here cognitive behaviour therapy consisted of providing education or a rationale for treatment, skills acquisition where palliative coping strategies like pacing an activity and deep muscle relaxation were taught, self-instructional training or guided practice in the generation and use of self-rewards, and a fourth application phase where patients practised these skills, reported back on their successes and failures and utilised their own individual thermal biofeedback units at home.

Comparing social support with biofeedback, Bradley *et al.* (1987) assigned chronic RA patients to five thermal biofeedback sessions or fifteen sessions of structured social support with family or friends. A comparison group was composed of those who had no additional contact with health professionals. The cognitive behaviour therapy group reported a significant reduction in pain and unpleasantness and showed less rheumatoid activity following treatment, indicating the superior effectiveness of biofeedback. However, both groups found the use of imagery and relaxation very helpful. While the results from this study do not give much immediate encouragement for the further use of social support with RA patients, Chapter 8 shows how varied definitions of social support can be and how other styles of support interventions might produce different conclusions.

Summary

In a recent major review, Parker *et al.* (1993) have concluded that cognitive behaviour therapy techniques are useful because they show improved health status for those with RA. Considering the outcome of nine studies which had used cognitive behaviour therapy techniques to treat adults with RA, they found that while many showed improvements at the end of treatment, most failed to sustain the benefits until follow-up. Furthermore, where improvement occurred, no single outcome measure was consistently sensitive to change; some studies found relief from pain, others saw improvements in emotional state, disability or disease activity. Many of the studies had some methodological limitation. The review reveals that cognitive behaviour therapy covers a very wide range of techniques. The absence of consensus about the quintessential components of a cognitive behaviour therapy programme is at present an impediment to the development of a streamlined programme which produces sustained benefits for RA patients.

Systematic maintenance in the form of regular and scheduled contact with patients following discharge has been a major strength of behaviour therapy techniques and contrasts with the conventional pattern of providing maintenance and support on the patient's request. In view of the poor results at follow-up from published cognitive behaviour therapy trials in this diagnostic group, Keefe and van Horn (1993) suggest that more attention should be paid to parrying relapse and to maintenance. Drawing on an interesting model by Marlatt and Gordon developed for smoking cessation, they show how cognitive behaviour therapy techniques and elements of educational programmes (see below) can be applied to intervene in those social and psychological processes which contribute to a major setback in therapy or a relapse. This useful model provides a new focus for research and should be taken seriously by those undertaking clinical work in this area.

SELF-EFFICACY AND PATIENT EDUCATION

Beliefs about control were discussed earlier and the concept of self-efficacy draws on this work in asking how far these beliefs are translated into actions because the person believes she is likely to be successful in what she does. Believing that you will succeed in opening a can of beans will encourage you to try, and this also applies to doing exercises to maintain a range of physical movement, controlling a diet or using an appliance.

The self-efficacy model provides a framework for understanding more about the behaviour of chronic pain patients inside and outside therapy (Bandura, 1974). Three dimensions have been proposed which may affect the ability to achieve a desired goal like pain relief. First, how difficult is the task expected to be? It is probable that the more difficult tasks will be avoided. Expectations are also affected by generality. While people may expect to perform a particular action successfully, their expectations about carrying out a broad range of activities may be quite different. Expectations also vary in strength; how confident are they about fulfilling their own expectations?

Self-efficacy has been used to explain actions taken to cope with pain as those with chronic painful diseases may believe that it is possible to control their pain and distress about illness. But how confident are they that they are capable of relieving it? Do they believe that they have the ability to exercise direct control over distressing painful events? Self-efficacy beliefs are being researched in the context of pain management and may help to explain why therapy is successful or not. Self-efficacy beliefs also affect patient adherence to medication (O'Leary, 1985). If perceptions of being self-efficacious rely on receiving medication, and medication is subsequently withdrawn, then strong self-efficacy beliefs may be rapidly dissipated (Bandura *et al.* 1987).

One problem with research in this area is the lack of consensus over self-efficacy measures. Lorig *et al.* (1989) have been developing a measure for use with arthritis patients which includes a comprehensive range of activities and symptoms. Typical items ask about whether you can walk 100 feet on flat ground in 20 seconds, or how certain you are that you can reduce your pain quite a bit. Items on fatigue, dealing with the frustration of arthritis, regulating activities, doing something to feel better when low, and comparisons with 'others like you' about how pain during activity is managed, provide a useful arthritis-centred measure. Unstable test–retest reliability results support Bandura's assertion that self-efficacy is not a personality dimension but a set of fluctuating beliefs and expectations about salient activities.

Bandura (1991) proposes three ways in which efficacy beliefs can bring relief from pain. Those who strongly believe they will be able to relieve their pain are more likely to seek out information and skills which will enable them to do this, and persist in doing them (O'Leary, 1985) and, conversely, those who believe they are less efficacious are likely to give up trying rapidly, if they are unsuccessful. Secondly, distressing expectations are reduced if a person feels self-efficacious. As distress encompasses anxiety and physical tension, it is possible to see how those with low self-efficacy beliefs may be more predisposed to greater discomfort. Thirdly, unpleasant sensations are more likely to be viewed as benign by those with strong beliefs in their self-efficacy and lack of fear about pain control has implications for lower pain levels. Bandura (1991) points out that those in pain draw on information stored in the memory about their own previous performances. Modelling and other vicarious learning add to these schemata. In short, 'nothing breeds success like success'.

People make inferences about their stamina – correct or otherwise – from internal physiological cues and Pennebaker (1982) has shown how ambiguous these bodily cues may be and for this reason they are open to substantial misinterpretation. To show how this happens for painful symptoms, Anderson & Pennebaker (1981) asked students to sign a consent form before taking part in an experiment which required them to place a finger on a piece of moving abrasive paper for one second. For one group of participants the words on the consent form said that they might feel some 'pain', for another group the word pain was replaced by 'pleasure' and the third control group did not read either word. The results confirmed that in line with the available schemata most of those in the pain group reported pain and those in the pleasure group pleasure. But when questioned during debriefing, members of both experimental groups denied that their sensations could possibly be interpreted in any alternative way. While the results of this study are not strong, it shows how ambiguous sensations can be and more importantly, the substantial influence of the context of these sensations in giving meaning to them. The implication here is that once the schemata are formed through the process of categorisation and labelling, it becomes difficult to alter these meanings. Such studies give insight into why the schemata that pain sufferers bring to cognitive therapy are so very resistant to change, particularly those where the reinterpretation of sensations is required.

But perhaps greater autonomic activity recorded from those with lower self-efficacy beliefs does provide them with some physiological feedback about coping. Those who hold higher self-efficacy beliefs are reported to be calmer as well as in more active control, and this appears to have direct implications for their autonomic activity (and vice versa). Evidence from a study by Bandura *et al.* (1988) supports the conclusion that the endogenous opioids blunt the aversive effects of stressors and influence people's ability to withstand pain. In particular it demonstrates the power of self-efficacy beliefs about pain control.

Also of relevance to the treatment of RA, strong self-efficacy beliefs have been shown to assist coping and to be associated with less functional disability and more problem-solving one year after treatment (Schiaffino *et al.,* 1991). Contrary to prediction, these investigations showed that if the pain was high, strong self-efficacy beliefs were related to greater depression a year later. The warning here is that depression may be the price that the self-efficacious pay if they are unsuccessful in controlling their pain in the long term. Such perceived failures deserve further investigation as it seems likely that different maintenance procedures will be required following the end of treatment to deal with the varied outcomes experienced by those with high and low self-efficacy beliefs.

In a review of the area, Bradley *et al.* (1984) conclude that RA appears to be particularly amenable to self-control training interventions and the promotion of self-care in those with RA is being explored using a variety of packages containing information, exercises and practice (Neuberger *et al.,* 1993). However, some studies have shown that the majority of people with RA already show moderate to high levels of positive and proactive self-care activity (Ailinger & Dear, 1993).

Patient education is one area where programmes have been established to improve self-efficacy. Lorig *et al.* (1987) reviewed seventy-six studies of education about arthritis published over a 10-year period, but only a third of these reported a significant change in knowledge. Of those showing some success (94 per cent of those that changed), the benefits were attributed to an increase in knowledge about the disease process or about treatment, or both. Practising exercises, joint-protection and relaxation improved pain, disability and other health indices. However, the effectiveness of patient education was little better than that reported for other arthritis treatments, such as the use of NSAIDs. More pertinent to the appraisal of self-efficacy, changes in behaviour were more often implied in studies than actually tested, and in the three studies where this test was carried out the association was not good. The most successful and more recent studies have tended to emphasise endurance exercise, encourage coping through self-efficacy and facilitate problem-solving. This daily routine of self-management shows more promise than the conventional programme of range-of-motion exercises and joint-protection activities carried out by physiotherapists.

Lorig's self-management course of six 2-hour sessions for twelve to eighteen participants is led by highly credible lay trainers who have personal experience of RA. They outline the physiology and pathology of the disease, create individual plans of exercises and relaxation and inform about nutrition and the appropriate use of joints. They also discuss medication use, solve medical problems and tackle communication problems encountered with the doctor. Reviewing the outcome of seventy-three courses which included more than 700 participants, Lorig *et al.* (1989) found a significant improvement in exercise frequency, relaxation methods and self-management knowledge 4 months after the end of the course. None of these changes was related to diagnosis. More specifically, reductions in pain were associated with doing more exercise.

More recent claims for the long-term benefits of self-management courses have been made by Lorig *et al.* (1993). Their review reports a significant reduction in several important outcome measures; pain was reduced on average by 20 per cent and subsequent visits to the doctor by 40 per cent, but despite an increase in activities, physical disability increased by 9 per cent. Furthermore the decline in pain persisted over 4 years, persuasively showing the relatively permanent effects of this type of self-care intervention programme. In the US, the savings for each patient with RA have been estimated at $648 (approximately £435). Based on these figures, national savings for the US alone could run into millions of dollars annually if self-management training was made widely available.

Such results underscore the overall picture emerging from a variety of psychological treatments directed at the relief of painful diseases, namely that psychological therapies take a long time to mature. Attitudes and beliefs rarely change overnight, and where people are using newly acquired techniques, they need time and opportunity to practise them properly and then to integrate them into their daily routine when they leave clinical care. Despite the current vogue for the economics of short-termism, there appear to be no short-cuts to creating and maintaining changes in beliefs and behaviour that will relieve disabling symptoms and endure. However, as with the menus of procedures available for cognitive behaviour therapy, it would be useful to know whether there are certain 'active ingredients' in these educational packages that are more efficacious than others. Such knowledge would lead to valuable streamlining of procedures and hence reductions in therapy time and costs accruing.

So should we be using behaviour therapy or education in the psychological treatment of people with RA? Assessing the results of published studies of cognitive behaviour therapy alone, from those where education is provided, Keefe and van Horn (1993) concluded that those which integrated the two treatments looked the most promising. Like other studies, they identified the most influential therapeutic components in this combination as self-efficacy, the use of pain-coping strategies and perceptions of control over pain. Directly tackling these key issues may turn out to be of more importance than using any specific therapy modality.

SUMMARY

Research to date indicates that there is considerable scope for the use of psychological therapies to relieve pain and assist disability in RA. However, there are several commonalities between the different techniques that are available and have been well researched. More progress is likely to be made if new approaches can be derived from recombining and assessing these tried and tested features in different packages rather than a continuing adherence to existing forms of therapy.

References

Achterberg-Lawlis, J. (1982) The psychological dimensions of arthritis, *Journal of Consulting and Clinical Psychology* 50(6): 984–92.

Achterberg, J., McGraw, P. and Lawlis, F.G. (1981) Rheumatoid arthritis: a study of relaxation and temperature biofeedback as an adjunctive therapy, *Biofeedback and Self-Regulation* 6(2): 207–23.

Affleck, G., Tennen, H., Urrows, S. and Higgins, P. (19xx) Individual differences in the day to day experience of chronic pain: a prospective daily study of rheumatoid arthritis patients, *Health Psychology* 10(6): 419–26.

Affleck, G., Tennen, H., Urrows, S. and Higgins, P. (1994) Person and contextual features of daily stress reactivity: individual differences in relations of undesirable daily events with mood disturbance in chronic pain intensity, *Journal of Personality and Social Psychology* 94: 329–60.

—— (1992) Neuroticism and the pain-mood relation in rheumatoid arthritis: insights from a prospective daily study, *Journal of Consulting and Clinical Psychology* 60(19): 119–26.

Affleck, G., Urrows, S., Tennen, H. and Higgins, P. (1992) Daily coping with pain from rheumatoid arthritis: patterns, and correlates, *Pain* 51: 221–9.

Affleck, G., Pfieffer, C., Tennen, H. and Fifield, J. (1987) Attributional processes in rheumatoid arthritis patients, *Arthritis and Rheumatism* 30(8): 927–31.

—— (1988) Social support and psychosocial adjustment to rheumatoid arthritis, *Arthritis Care and Research* 1: 71–7.

Affleck, G., Tennen, H., Pfeiffer, C. and Fifield, J. (1987) Appraisals of control and predictability in adapting to a chronic disease, *Journal of Personality and Social Psychology* 53(2): 273–9.

Affleck, G., Tennen, H., Pfeiffer, C., Fifield, J., and Rowe, J. (1987) Downward social comparison and coping with serious medical problems, *American Journal of Orthopsychiatry* 57: 570–8.

Agras, W.S. (1989) Understanding compliance with the medical regimen: the scope of the problem and a theoretical perspective, *Arthritis Care and Research* 2: S2–7.

Ahles, T.A., Yunus, M.B., Gaulier, B., Riley, S.D. and Masi, A.T. (1986) The use of contemporary norms in the study of chronic pain patients, *Pain* 24: 159–63.

Ahlmen, M., Sullivan, M. and Bjelle, A. (1988) Team versus non-team outpatient care in rheumatoid arthritis, *Arthritis & Rheumatism* 31: 471–9.

Aho, K., Koskenvuo, M., Tuominen, J. and Kaprio, J. (1986) Occurrence of rheumatoid arthritis in a nationwide series of twins, *Journal of Rheumatology* 13: 899–902.

Ailinger, R.L. and Dear, M.R. (1993) Self care agency in persons with rheumatoid arthritis, *Arthritis Care and Research* 6(3): 134–40.

Akehurst, R. (1992) An evaluation of the cost of arthritis, *British Journal of Medical Economics* 5: v–vi.

Anderson, J., Felson, D., Meenan, R. *et al.* (1990) Secular trends in rheumatoid arthritis trials, *Arthritis and Rheumatism* 33 (suppl.): S138–90.

Anderson, A.D. and Pennebaker, J.W. (1981) Pain and pleasure, *European Journal of Social Psychology* 10: 207–12.

Anderson, J., Firschein, H. and Meenan, R. (1989) Sensitivity of a health status measure to short-term clinical changes in arthritis, *Arthritis & Rheumatism* 32: 844–50.

Anderson, K., Bradley, L., Turner, R., Agudelo, C., Pisko, E., Salley, A. and Fletcher, K. (1992) Observation of pain behaviour in Rheumatoid Arthritis patients during physical examination; relationship to disease activity and psychological variables, *Arthritis Care and Research* 5(1): 49–56.

Anderson, K., Bradley, L., Young, L., McDaniel, L. and Wise, C. (1985) Rheumatoid arthritis: review of psychological factors related to etiology, effects and treatment, *Psychological Bulletin* 98: 350–7.

Anderson, R. and Bury, M. (1988) *Living with Chronic Illness: The Experience of Patients and their Families*, London: Unwin Hyman.

Anderson, W.T. and Helm, D.T. (1979). The physician–patient encounter: a process of reality negotiation, in E.G. Jaco (ed.), *Patients, physicians, and illness*, New York: Free Press, pp. 259–71.

Antonovsky, A. (1979) *Health, Stress, and Coping*, London: Jossey-Bass.

Antonucci, T.A. (1985) Social support: theoretical advances, recent findings and pressing issues, in I.G. Sarason, B.R. Sarason (eds.), *Social Support: Theory, Research and Applications*, Dordrecht, The Netherlands: Martinus Nijhoff, pp. 21–37.

Arber, S. (1990) Revealing women's health: re-analyzing the General Household Survey, in H. Roberts (ed.), *Women's Health Counts*, London: Routledge.

Arluke, A. (1980) Judging drugs: patients' conceptions of therapeutic efficacy in the treatment of arthritis, *Human Organization* 39: 84–7.

Armitage, K.J., Schneiderman, L.J. and Bass, R.A. (1979) Responses of physicians to medical complaints in men and women, *Journal of the American Medical Association* 241: 2168–87.

Arnett, F.C., Edworthy, S.M., Bloch, D.A. *et al.* (1988) The American Rheumatism Association revised criteria for the classification of rheumatoid arthritis, *Arthritis and Rheumatism* 31: 315–24.

Arnett, F., Edworthy, S., Bloch, D. *et al.* (1987) The American Rheumatism Association 1987 revised criteria for classification of

rheumatoid arthritis, *Arthritis and Rheumatism* 31: 315–24.
Arthritis Care (1989) *Arthritis: The Painful Challenge*, London: Arthritis Care.
Ash, G. (1992) Depression in arthritis patients, in 'Arthritis and the Psyche'. Conference Proceedings, No. 9. Arthritis and Rheumatism Council of Great Britain.
Badley, E.M. (1991) Population projections and the effect on rheumatology, *Annals of the Rheumatic Diseases* 50: 3–6.
Badley, E.M. (1992) The impact of musculoskeletal disorders on the Canadian population, *Journal of Rheumatology* 19: 337–40.
Badley, E.M. and Papageorgiou, A.C. (1989) Visual analogue scales as a measure of pain in arthritis: a study of overall pain and pain in individual joints, at rest and on movement, *Journal of Rheumatology* 16(1):102.
Badley, E.M. and Wood, P.H.N. (1979) Attitudes of the public to arthritis, *Annals of the Rheumatic Diseases* 38: 97–100.
Baker, G.H.B. (1981) Psychological management, *Clinics in Rheumatic Diseases* 7: 455–67.
Baker, R.R. (1984) Attitudes of health care providers toward elderly patients with normal aging and disease-related symptoms, *The Gerontologist* 24: 543–45.
Balaban, D., Fagi, P., Goldfarb, N. and Nettler, S. (1986) Weights for scoring the quality of well-being instrument among rheumatoid arthritics, *Medical Care* 24: 973–80.
Bandura, A. (1974) Behaviour theory and models of man, *American Psychologist* 29 (12): 859–69.
Bandura, A. (1991) Self efficiency mechanisms in physiological activation and health promoting behaviour, in J. Madden (ed.) *Neurobiology of Learning, Emotion and Affect*, New York: Raven Press, pp. 229–69.
Bandura, A., Cloffi, D., Taylor, C.B. and Brouillard, M.E. (1988) Perceived self-efficacy in coping with cognitive stressors and opioid activation, *Journal of Personality and Social Psychology* 55: 479–88.
Bandura, A., O'Leary, A., Taylor, C.B., Gauthier, J. and Gossard, D. (1987) Perceived self-efficacy and path control – opioid and non-opioid mechanisms, *Journal of Personality and Social Psychology* 53 (3): 563–71.
Barnes, C.G. and Mason, M. (1975) Rheumatoid arthritis, in M. Mason and H.L.F. Curry (eds), *Introduction to clinical rheumatology*, Bath: Pitman, ch. 2.
Barrera, M. Jr. (1986) Distinctions between social support concepts, measures and models, *American Journal of Community Psychology* 14: 413–45.
Becker, M. (1985) Patient adherence to prescribed therapies, *Medical Care* 23: 539–55.
Beckham, J.C., Keefe, F. *et al.* (1991) Pain coping strategies in rheumatoid arthritis, *Behavioral Therapy* 22: 113–24.
Beecher, H.K. (1956) Relationship of the significance of wound to pain experienced. *Journal of the American Medical Association* 161(17): 1609–1613.
Belcon, M.C., Haynes, B. and Tugwell, P. (1984) A critical review of compliance studies in rheumatoid arthritis, *Arthritis and Rheumatism*

27: 1227–33.

Ben-Sira, Z. (1976) The function of the professional's affective behavior in client satisfaction: a revised approach to social interaction theory, *Journal of Health and Social Behavior* 17: 3–11.

— (1980) Affective and instrumental components in the physician–patient relationship: an additional dimension of interaction theory, *Journal of Health and Social Behavior* 21: 170–80.

— (1985) Primary medical care and coping with stress and disease: the inclination of primary care practitioners to demonstrate affective behaviour, *Social Science and Medicine* 21: 485–98.

Bensing, J.M., Van der Brink-Muinen, A. & de Bakker, D.H. (1993) Gender differences in practice style: a Dutch study of general practitioners, *Medical Care* 31: 219–29.

Bergner, M., Bobbitt, R., Carter, W. and Gilson, B. (1981) The Sickness Impact Profile: development and final revision of a health status measure, *Medical Care* 19: 787–805.

Berkman, L.F. (1985) The relationship of social networks and social support to morbidity and mortality, in S. Cohen & S.L. Syme (eds), *Social support and health*, NY: Academic (pp. 243–62).

Bernstein, B. & Kane, R. (1981) Physicians' attitudes toward female patients, *Medical Care* 19: 600–8.

Bijlsma, J.W.J., Huiskes, C. *et al.* (1991) Relation between patients' own health assessment and clinical and laboratory findings in rheumatoid arthritis, *Journal of Rheumatology* 18: 650–3.

Billings, A.G. and Moos, R.H. (1984) Coping, stress and social resources amongst adults with unipolar depression, *Journal of Personality and Social Psychology* 46: 877–91.

Binstock, R.H. (1983) The aged as scapegoat, *The Gerontologist* 23: 136–43.

Birkel, R.C. and Reppucci, N.D. (1983) Social networks, information-seeking, and the utilization of services, *American Journal of Community Psychology* 11: 185–206.

Blalock, S.J., DeVellis, B.M., DeVellis, R.F., Giorgio, K.B., Van H. Sauter, S., Jordan, J.M., Keefe, F.J. and Mutrain, E.J. (1993) Psychological well-being among people with recently diagnosed rheumatoid arthritis: do self perceptions of abilities make a difference? *Arthritis Care and Research*.

Blalock, S., DeVellis, R. et al. (1992) Coping with rheumatoid arthritis: is one problem the same as another?, *Arthritis and Rheumatism* 00:000.

Blalock, S.J., and DeVellis, R.F. (1992) Rheumatoid arthritis and depression: an overview, *Bulletin of Rheumatic Disease* 41(1): 6–8.

Blalock, S.J., DeVellis, R. et al. (1989) Validity of the Centre for Epidemiological Studies Depression Scale in Arthritis Populations, *Arthritis and Rheumatism* 32(8): 991–7.

Blalock, S.J., DeVellis, R.F., DeVellis, B.M. (1989) Social comparisons among individuals with rheumatoid arthritis, *Journal of Applied Social Psychology* 19: 665–80.

Blaxter, M. (1983) The causes of disease: women talking, *Social Science and Medicine* 17: 58–69.

Bloom, S.W. (1963) *The Doctor and his Patient*, New York: Free Press.

Bombardier, C., Ware, J., Russell, U., Larson, M., Chalmers, A., Read, J. and Auranofin Cooperating Group (1986) Auranofin therapy and quality of life in patients with rheumatoid arthritis, *American Journal of Medicine* 81: 565–78.

Bradley, L.A. (1989a) Psychosocial factors and disease outcomes in rheumatoid arthritis: old problems, new solutions, and a future agenda, *Arthritis and Rheumatism* 32(12): 1611–14.

—— (1989b) Adherence with treatment regimens among adult rheumatoid arthritis patients: current status and future directions, *Arthritis Care and Research* 2: S33–9.

Bradley, L.A., Young, L.D., Anderson, K.O., Turner, R.A., Agudelo, C.A., McDaniel, L.K., Pisko, E.J., Semble, E.L. and Morgan, T.M. (1987) Effects of psychological therapy on pain behaviour of rheumatoid arthritis patients: treatment, outcome and six-month follow-up, *Arthritis and Rheumatism* 30(10): 1105–14.

Bradley, L.A., Turner, R.A., Young, L.D., Agudelo, C.A., Anderson, K.O. and McDaniel, L.K. (1985) Effects of cognitive-behavioural therapy on pain behaviour of rheumatoid arthritis patients: preliminary outcomes, *Scandinavian Journal of Behavioural Medicine* 14: 51–64.

Bradley, L.A., Young, L.D., Anderson, K.O., McDaniel, L.K., Turner, R.A. and Agudelo, C.A. (1984) Psychological approaches to the management of arthritis pain, *Social Science and Medicine* 19(12): 1353–60.

Briscoe, M. (1982) Sex differences in psychological well-being, *Psychological Medicine Monograph Number 1*, Cambridge: Cambridge University Press.

Brody, E.M. (1989) The family at risk, in E. Light & B.D. Lebowitz (eds) *Alzheimer's disease treatment and family stress: directions for research*, Rockville, MD: US Department of Health and Human Services, pp. 2–49.

Brook, A. and Corbett, M. (1971) Radiographic change in early rheumatoid disease, *Annals of Rheumatic Diseases* 36: 71–3.

Brooks, B., Jordan, J., Divinew, G., Smith, K. and Neelon, F. (1990) The impact of psychologic factors on measurement of functional status, *Medical Care* 28: 793–804.

Brooks, P. (1993) Clinical management of rheumatoid arthritis, *Lancet* 341: 286–90.

Brown, G.K., Nicassio, P. *et al.* (1989) Pain coping strategies and depression in rheumatoid arthritis, *Journal of Consultative Clinical Psychology* 57: 652–7.

Brown, G.K., Wallston, K.A. and Nicassio, P.M. (1989) Social support and depression in rheumatoid arthritis: a one-year prospective study, *Journal of Applied Social Psychology* 19: 1164–81.

Brown, G.K. and Nicassio, P.M. (1987) Development of a questionnaire for the assessment of active and passive coping strategies in chronic pain patients, *Pain* 31: 53–63.

Bruhn, J.G. and Philips, B.U. (1984) Measuring social support: a synthesis of current approaches, *Journal of Behavioral Medicine*, 7: 151–69.

Buckley, L.M., Vacek, P., Cooper, S.M. (1990) Educational and psychosocial needs of patients with chronic disease: a survey of preferences of patients with rheumatoid arthritis, *Arthritis Care and Research* 3: 5–10.

Burckhart, C. (1985) The impact of arthritis on quality of life, *Nursing Research* 34: 11–16.

Bury, M.R. (1982) Chronic illness as biographical disruption, *Sociology of Health and Illness* 4: 167–82.

—— (1985) Arthritis in the family: problems in adaptation and self-care, in N.M. Hadler and D.B. Gillings (eds), *Arthritis in society: the impact of musculo-skeletal diseases*, London: Butterworth.

—— (1988) Meanings at risk: the experience of arthritis, in R. Anderson and M.R. Bury (eds), *Living with Chronic Illness: The Experience of Patients and their Families*, London: Unwin Hyman, pp. 89–116.

—— (1991) The sociology of chronic illness: a review of research and prospects, *Sociology of Health and Illness* 14: 451–68.

Bury, M.R. and Wood, P.H.N. (1978) Sociological perspectives in research on disablement, *International Rehabilitation Medicine* 1: 25–32.

Callahan, L., Bloch, D. and Pincus, T. (1992) Identification of work disability in rheumatoid arthritis, *Journal of Clinical Epidemiology* 45: 127–38.

Calnan, M. (1987) *Health and Illness: the Lay Perspective*, London: Tavistock.

Campbell, J.N., Raja, S.N., Cohen, R.H., Manning, D.C., Khan, A.A. and Meyer, R.A. (1989) Peripheral neural mechanisms of nociception, in P.D. Wall and R. Melzack (eds), *Textbook of Pain*, second edition, Edinburgh: Churchill Livingston, pp. 22–45.

Caruso, I., Santandrea, S., Puttini, P., *et al.* (1990) Clinical laboratory and radiographic features in early rheumatoid arthritis, *Journal of Rheumatology* 17: 1263–7.

Carvalho, A., Graudal, H. and Jorgensen, B. (1980) Evaluation of the progression of rheumatoid arthritis, *Acta Radiologica (Diagnosis)* 4: 545–50.

Carver, C.S., Scheier, M.F. *et al.* (1989) Assessing coping strategies: a theoretically based approach, *Journal of Personality and Social Psychology*, 56: 267–83.

Cassileth, B., Lusk, E., Strouse, T., Miller, D., Brown, L., Cross, P. and Tenaglia, A. (1984) Psychosocial status in chronic illness: a comparative analysis of six diagnostic groups, *New England Journal of Medicine* 311: 506–11.

Cella, D. and Tulsky, D. (1990) Measuring quality of life today: methodological aspects, *Oncology* 4: 29–38.

Chalmers, A. (1984) Belief systems – patient and physician views of arthritis and its treatment (editorial), *Journal of Rheumatology* 11: 1–2.

Chambers, L., MacDonald, L., Tugwell, P., Buchanan, W. and Kraag, G. (1982) The McMaster Health Index Questionnaire as a measure of quality of life for patients with rheumatoid disease, *Journal of Rheumatology* 9: 780–4.

Chrisman, N. (1977) The health seeking process: an approach to the natural history of illness, *Culture, Medicine and Psychiatry* 1: 351–77.

Cilberto, D.J., Levin, J. and Arluke, A. (1981) Nurses' diagnostic stereotyping of the elderly, *Research on Aging* 3: 299–310.

Cohen, F. (ed.) (1987) *Measurement of Coping*. Stress and Health: Issues in Research Methodology, California: John Wiley and Sons Ltd.

Cohen, F. and Lazarus, R. (1973) Active coping processes, coping dispositions and recovery from surgery, *Psychosomatic Medicine*, 35: 375–89.

Cohen, S. (1988) Psychosocial models of the role of social support in the etiology of physical disease, *Health Psychology*, 7: 269–97.

Cohen, S. and Wills, T.A. (1985) Stress, social support, and the buffering hypothesis, *Psychological Bulletin*, 98: 310–57.

Colameco, S., Becker, L.A. and Simpson, M. (1983) Sex bias in the assessment of patients' complaints, *Journal of Family Practice* 16: 1117–21.

Comaroff, J. and Maguire, P. (1981) Ambiguity and the search for meaning: childhood leukaemia in the modern clinical context, *Social Science and Medicine* 15b: 115–23.

Comstock, L.M., Hooper, E.M., Goodwin, J.M. and Goodwin, J.S. (1982) Physician behaviors that correlate with patient satisfaction, *Journal of Medical Education* 57: 105–12.

Conant, E.B. (1983) Addressing patients by their first names, *New England Journal of Medicine* 308: 226.

Conn, D.L. (1993) The doctor speaks: we have to trust each other, *Arthritis Today*, 7 (6): 24–6.

Corbin, J. and Strauss, A. (1988) *Unending work and care: managing chronic illness at home*, London: Jossey-Bass.

Cox, D., Fitzpatrick, R., Fletcher, A., Gore, S., Spiegelhalter, D. and Jones, D. (1992) Quality of life assessment: can we keep it simple? *Journal of the Royal Statistical Society* 155: 353–93.

Coyne, J.C., Ellard, J.H. and Smith, D.A.F. (1990) Social support, interdependence, and the dilemmas of helping, in B.R. Sarason, I.G. Sarason & G.R. Pierce (eds), *Social support: an interactional view*, New York: Wiley, pp. 129–49.

Coyne, J.C., Wortman, C.B., Lehman, D. (1988) The other side of support: emotional overinvolvement, and miscarried helping, in B.H. Gottlieb (ed.), *Social support: formats, processes, and effects*, Newbury Park, CA: Sage Publications pp. 305–30.

Coyne, J.C., and DeLongis, A. (1986) Going beyond social support: the role of social relationships in adaptation, *Journal of Consulting and Clinical Psychology*, 54: 454–60.

Creed, F. (1990) Psychological disorders in rheumatoid arthritis: a growing consensus? *Annals of the Rheumatic Diseases* 49: 808–12.

Cronan, T.A., Kaplan, R.M. and Kozin, F. (1993) Factors affecting unprescribed remedy use among people with self reported arthritis, *Arthritis Care and Research* 6 (3) 149–55.

Cronan, T.A., Kaplan, R.M., Posner, L. Blumberg, E., Kozin, F. (1989) Prevalence of the use of unconventional remedies for arthritis in a metropolitan community, *Arthritis and Rheumatism* 32: 1604–7.

Crown, S., Crown, J.M. and Fleming, A. (1975) Aspects of the psychology and epidemiology of rheumatoid disease, *Psychological Medicine* 5: 291–9.

Cunningham, L. and Kelsey, J. (1984) Epidemiology of muskuloskeletal impairments and associated disability, *American Journal of Public Health* 74: 574–9.

Cutrona, C.E., Russell, D.W. (1990) Type of social support and specific stress: toward a theory of optimal matching, in I.G. Sarason & B.R. Sarason (eds), *Social Support: An Interactional View*, New York: Wiley, pp. 319–66.

Daltroy, L.H. (1993) Doctor–patient communication in rheumatological disorders, in S. Newman & M. Shipley (eds), *Psychological Aspects of Rheumatic Disease. Ballière's Clinical Rheumatology*, 7 (2): 221–40. London: Baillière Tindall.

Daltroy, L.H. and Godin, G. (1989) Spouse intention to encourage cardiac patients' participation in exercise, *American Journal of Health Promotion* 4: 12–17.

Da Silva, J. and Hall, G. (1992) Effects of gender and sex hormones, in D. Scott (ed.), *Baillière's Clinical Rheumatology: The Course and Outcome of Rheumatoid Arthritis*, London: Baillière Tindall, 193–220.

Davey Smith, G. and Egger, M. (1993) Socioeconomic differentials in wealth and health. *British Medical Journal* 307: 1085–6.

Dawes, P. and Symmons, D. (1992) Short-term effects of antirheumatic drugs, in D. Scott (ed.), *Baillière's Clinical Rheumatology: The Course and Outcome of Rheumatoid Arthritis*, London: Baillière Tindall, pp. 117–40.

Deighton, C., Surtees, D. and Walker, D. (1992) Influence of the severity of rheumatoid arthritis on sex differences in Health Assessment Questionnaire scores, *Annals of Rheumatic Diseases*, 51: 473–5.

Delbanco, T.L. (1992) Enriching the doctor–patient relationship by inviting the patient's perspective, *Annals of Internal Medicine* 116: 414–18.

DeVellis, B.M. (1993) Depression in rheumatological diseases, in S. Newman & M. Shipley (eds) *Psychological Aspects of Rheumatic Disease*. *Baillière's Clinical Rheumatology*, 7 (2): 241–58. London: Baillière Tindal.

Deyo, R.A. (1982) Compliance with therapeutic regimens in arthritis: issues, current status, and a future agenda, *Seminars in Arthritis and Rheumatism* 12: 233–44.

—— (1988) Measuring the quality of life of patients with rheumatoid arthritis, in *Quality of life: assessment and application*, S.R. Walker and R.M. Rosser (eds), Lancaster: MTP Press, p. 205.

Deyo, R.A. (1990) Measuring the quality of life of patients with Rheumatoid Arthritis, in R.A. Sternbach (ed.) *The Psychology of Pain*, New York: Raven Press.

Deyo, R. and Centor, R. (1986) Assessing the responsiveness of functional scales to clinical change: an analogy to diagnostic test performance, *Journal of Chronic Diseases* 39: 897–906.

Deyo, R. and Inui, T. (1984) Towards clinical applications of health status measures: sensitivity of scales to clinically important changes, *Health Services Research* 19: 275–89.

Deyo, R., Inui, T., Leininger, J. and Overman, S. (1983) Measuring functional outcomes in chronic disease: a comparison of traditional scales and a self-administered health status questionnaire in patients with rheumatoid arthritis, *Medical Care* 21: 180–92.

—— (1982) Physical and psychosocial function in rheumatoid arthritis, *Archives of Internal Medicine* 142: 879–82.

Deyo, R.A., Inui, T.S. and Sullivan, B. (1981) Noncompliance with arthritis drugs: magnitude, correlates, and clinical implications, *Journal of Rheumatology* 8: 931–6.

DiMatteo, M.D. & DiNicola, D.D. (1982) Social science and the art of medicine: from Hippocrates to holism, in H.S. Friedman & M.R. DiMatteo (eds), *Interpersonal Issues in Health Care*, New York: Academic Press, pp. 9–31.

DiMatteo, M.R. and Hays, R. (1981) Social support and serious illness, in B.H. Gottlieb (eds), *Social Networks and Social Support*, Beverly Hills, CA: Sage, pp. 117–48.

—— (1984) Toward a more therapeutic physician–patient relationship, in S.W. Duck (ed.), *Personal Relationships 5: Repairing Personal Relationships*, London: Academic Press, pp. 1–20.

DiNicola, D.D. and DiMatteio, M.D. (1984) Practitioners, patients and compliance with medial regimens, in A. Baum, S.E. Taylor and J.E. Singer (eds), *Handbook of Psychology and Health*, Hillsdale, NJ. Embaum, vol. 4, pp. 55–84.

Dohrenwend, B.S., Dohrenwend, B.P., Dodson, M. and Shrout, P.E. (1984) Symptoms, hassles, social supports and life events: problems of confounded measures, *Journal of Abnormal Psychology* 93: 222–30.

Donovan, J.L., Blake, D.R. and Fleming, W.G. (1989) The patient is not a blank sheet: lay beliefs and their relevance to patient education, *British Journal of Rheumatology* 28: 58–61.

Downie, R. (1992) Healthcare ethics and casuistry (editorial), *Journal of Medical Ethics* 18(2): 61–2.

Dubner, R. (1989) Methods of assessing pain in animals, in P.D. Wall and R. Melzack (eds), *Textbook of Pain*, second edition, Edinburgh: Churchill Livingston, pp. 247–56.

Dugowson, C., Koepsell, T., Voight, L. *et al.* (1991) Rheumatoid arthritis in women: incidence rates in a group health cooperative, Seattle Washington 1987–9, *Arthritis and Rheumatism* 34: 1502–7.

Dunbar, J., Dunning, E.J., Dwyer, K. (1989) Compliance measurement with arthritis regimen, *Arthritis Care and Research* 2: S8–S16.

Dunkel-Schetter, C. (1984) Social support and cancer: findings based on patient interviews and their implications, *Journal of Social Issues* 40: 77–98.

Dunkel-Schetter, C., Feinstein, L.G., Taylor, S.E., Falke, R.L. (1992) Patterns of coping with cancer, *Health Psychology* 11: 79–87.

Dunkel-Schetter, C., Bennett, T.L. (1990) Differentiating the cognitive and behavioral aspects of social support, in B.R. Sarason, I.G. Sarason and G.R. Pierce (eds), *Social support: an interactional view*, New York: John Wiley & Sons, pp. 267–96.

Dunkel-Schetter, C., Folkman, S. *et al.* (1987) Correlates of social support

receipt, *Journal of Personality and Social Psychology* 53: 71–80.
Dunkel-Schetter, C. and Wortman, C.B. (1982) The interpersonal dynamics of cancer, in H.S. Friedman & M.R. DiMatteo (eds), *Interpersonal issues in health care*, New York: Academic Press, pp. 69–100.
Earle, J., Perricone, P., Maultsby, D., Pericone, N., Turner, R. and Davis, J. (1979) Psycho-social adjustment of rheumatoid arthritis patients from two alternative treatment settings, *Journal of Rheumatology* 6: 80–7.
Eckenrode, J. (1991) Introduction and overview, *The Social Context of Coping*. New York: Plenum Press, pp. 1–12.
Eckenrode, J. and Gore, S. (1981) Stressful life events and social support: the significance of context, in B.H. Gottlieb (ed), *Social Networks and Social Support*, Beverly Hills, CA: Sage, pp. 43–68.
Ekdahl, C., Eberhardt, K., Andersson, S. and Svensson, B. (1988) Assessing disability in patients with rheumatoid arthritis, *Scandinavian Journal of Rheumatology* 17: 263–71.
Elder, R.G. (1973) Social class and lay explanations for the etiology of arthritis, *Journal of Health and Social Behaviour* 14: 28–38.
Endler, N.S. and Parker, J. (1990a) Multidimensional assessment of coping: a critical evaluation, *Journal of Personality and Social Psychology* 58: 844–54.
—(1990b) *Coping Inventory for Stressful Situations (CISS) manual*, Toronto: Multi-Health Systems.
Engel, A. (1968) Rheumatoid arthritis in US adults 1960–62, in P.H. Bennett and P.H.N. Wood (eds), *Population Studies of the Rheumatic Diseases*, Amsterdam: Excerpta Medica.
Engel, G.L. (1977) The need for a new medical model: a challenge for biomedicine, *Science* 196: 129–36.
Feinberg, J. (1988) The effect of patient–practitioner interaction on compliance: a review of the literature and application in rheumatoid arthritis, *Patient Education and Counseling*, 11: 171–87.
Felson, D., Anderson, J., Boers, M. *et al.* (1993) The American College of Rheumatology preliminary core set of disease activity measures for rheumatoid arthritis clinical trials, *Arthritis and Rheumatism* 36: 729–40.
Felson, D., Anderson, J. and Meenan, R. (1990) The comparative efficacy and toxicity of second-line drugs in rheumatoid arthritis, *Arthritis and Rheumatism* 33: 1449–61.
Felton, B.J. (1990) Coping and social support in older people's experiences of chronic illness, in M.A.P. Stevens and S. Hobfoll (eds), *Stress and Coping in Late Life Families*, Washington DC: Hemisphere, pp. 153–71.
Felton, B. and Revenson, T.A. (1987) Age differences in coping with chronic illness, *Psychology and Aging* 2: 164–70.
Felton, B.J., Revenson, T.A. and Hinrichsen, G.A. (1984) Stress and coping in the explanation of psychological adjustment among chronically ill adults, *Social Sciences and Medicine* 18(10): 889–98.
Ferguson, K. and Bole, G.G. (1979) Family support, health beliefs and therapeutic compliance in patients with rheumatoid arthritis, *Patient Counselling and Health Education* (Winter/Spring): 101–5.

Fernandez, E. and Turk, D.C. (1989) The utility of cognitive coping strategies for altering pain perception: a meta-analysis, *Pain* 38(2): 123–35.

Fifield, J., Reisine, S. and Grady, K. (1991) Work disability and the experience of pain and depression in rheumatoid arthritis, *Social Science and Medicine* 33: 579–86.

Fitzgerald, M. (1989) Arthritis and the nervous system, *Trends in Neuroscience* 12: 86–7.

Fitzpatrick, R. (1989) Lay concepts of illness, in P. Brown (ed), *Perspectives in Medical Sociology*, Belmont, California: Wadsworth.

Fitzpatrick, R., Fletcher, A., Gore, S., Jones D., Spieglehalter, D. and Cox, D. (1992) Quality of life measures in health care. I: Applications and issues in assessment, *British Medical Journal* 305: 1074–77.

Fitzpatrick, R., Newman, S., Archer, R. and Shipley, M. (1991) Social support, disability and depression: a longitudinal study of RA, *Social Science and Medicine* 33: 605–11.

Fitzpatrick, R., Newman, S., Lamb, R. and Shipley, M. (1988) Social relationships and psychological well-being in rheumatoid arthritis, *Social Science and Medicine* 27: 399–403.

—— (1989) A comparison of measures of health status in rheumatoid arthritis, *British Journal of Rheumatology* 28: 201–6

—— (1990) Helplessness and control in rheumatoid arthritis, *International Journal of Health Sciences* 1: 17–24.

Fitzpatrick, R., Ziebland, S., Jenkinson, C., Mowat, A. and Mowat, A. (1991) The social dimension of health status measures in rheumatoid arthritis, *International Disability Studies* 13: 34–7.

—— (1992) A generic health status instrument in the assessment of rheumatoid arthritis, *British Journal of Rheumatology* 31: 87–90.

—— (1993a) A comparison of the sensitivity to change of several health status instruments in rheumatoid arthritis, *Journal of Rheumatology* 20: 429–36.

—— (1993b) Transition questions to assess outcomes in rheumatoid arthritis, *British Journal of Rheumatology* 32: 807–11.

Fleming, A., Crown, J. and Corbett, M. (1976) Early rheumatoid arthritis, *Annals of Rheumatic Diseases* 35: 357–60.

Flor, H. and Turk, D.C. (1988) Chronic back pain and rheumatoid arthritis: predicting pain and disability from cognitive variables, *Journal of Behavioural Medicine* 11(3) 251–65.

Folkman, S. and Lazarus, R. (1980) An analysis of coping in a middle-aged community sample, : 219–39.

—— (1985) If it changes it must be a process. Study of emotion and coping during three stages of college examination, *Journal of Personality and Social Psychology* 48: 150–70.

—— (1988) *Manual for the Ways of Coping Questionnaire*, Palo Alto: Consulting Psychologists Press.

Folkman, S., Lazarus, R.S. *et al.* (1986) The dynamics of a stressful encounter: cognitive appraisal, coping and encounter outcomes, *Journal of Personality and Social Psychology* 50: 992–1003.

Folkman, S., Lazraus, R. *et al.* (1987) Age differences in stress and coping, 2: 171–84.

Fordyce, W.E. (1976) *Behavioural Methods for Chronic Pain and Illness*, St Louis, Miss.: Mosby.
Fordyce, W.E. (1988) Pain and suffering: a reappraisal, *American Psychologist* 43(4): 276–83.
Forsterling, F. (1985) Attributional retraining: a review, *Psychological Bulletin* 98(3): 495–512.
Foster, G. (1976) Disease etiologies in non-Western medical systems, *American Anthropologist* 78: 773–82.
Frank, R., Beck, N., Parker, J., Kashani, J., Elliott, T., Haut, A., Smith, E., Atwood, C., Brownlee-Duffeck, M. and Kay, D. (1988) Depression in rheumatoid arthritis, *Journal of Rheumatology* 15: 920–5.
Frankel, S. (1991) The epidemiology of indications, *Journal of Epidemiology and Community Health* 45: 257–9.
Friedman, H.S. (1982) Nonverbal communication in medical interaction, in H.S. Friedman and M.R. DiMatteo (eds), *Interpersonal Issues in Health Care*, New York: Academic Press, pp. 51–6.
Friedman, L.C., Nelson, D.V. *et al.* (1992) The relationship of dispositional optimism, daily life stress, and domestic environment to coping methods used by cancer patients, *Journal of Behavioural Medicine* 15: 127–41.
Fries, J.F. (1979) *Arthritis: a comprehensive guide*. New York: Addison Wesley.
Fries, J., Spitz, P. and Young, D. (1982) The dimensions of health outcomes: the Health Assessment Questionnaire, disability and pain scales, *Journal of Rheumatology* 9: 789–93.
Gabe, J., Kelleher, D. and Williams, G.H. (eds) (1994) *Challenging Medicine*, London: Routledge.
Gardiner, B. (1980) Psychological aspects of rheumatoid arthritis, *Psychological Medicine* 10 (1): 159–63.
Gardiner, P., Sykes, H.A., Hassey, G. and Walker, D. (1993) An evaluation of the Health Assessment Questionnaire in long term longitudinal follow-up of disability in rheumatoid arthritis, *British Journal of Rheumatology* 32: 724–8.
Gaston-Johansson, F. and Gustafsson, M. (1990) Rheumatoid arthritis: determination of pain characteristics and comparison of RAI and VAS in its measurement, *Pain* 41: 35–40.
Geersten, H.R., Gray, R.M. and Ward, J.R. (1973) Patient non-compliance within the context of seeking medical care for arthritis, *Journal of Chronic Diseases* 26: 689–98.
Gibson, T. and Clark, B. (1985) Use of simple analgesics in rheumatoid arthritis, *Annals of Rheumatic Diseases* 44: 27–9.
Goffman, E. (1972) *Encounters*, Harmondsworth: Penguin.
Goldenberg, D.L. (1987) Fibromyalgia syndrome: an emerging but controversial condition, *Journal of the American Medical Association* 257.
Goodenow, C., Reisine, S.T. and Grady, K.E. (1990) Quality of social support and associated social and psychological functioning in women with rheumatoid arthritis, *Health Psychology* 9: 266–84.
Gore, S. (1981) Stress-buffering functions of social support: an appraisal and clarification of research models, in B.S. Dohrenwend and B.P.

Dohrenwend (eds), *Stressful Life Events and their Contexts,* New York: Prodist, pp. 202–22.
Gottlieb, B.H. (1983) *Social Support Strategies: Guidelines for Mental Health Practice*, Beverly Hills, CA: Sage.
— (ed.) (1988) *Marshalling Social Support*, Beverly Hills, CA: Sage.
Gove, W. and Tudor, J. (1973) Adult sex roles and mental illness, *American Journal of Sociology* 77: 812–35.
Gray, D. (1983) 'Arthritis': variation in beliefs about joint disease, *Medical Anthropology* 7: 29–46.
Greene, M.G., Hoffman, S., Charon, R. and Adelman, R. (1987) Psychosocial concerns in the medical encounter: a comparison of the interactions of doctors with their old and young patients, *The Gerontologist* 27: 164–8.
Grennan, D.M. and Jayson, M.I.V. (1989) Rheumatoid arthritis, in P.D. Wall and R. Melzack (eds) *Textbook of Pain*, Second edition, Edinburgh: Churchill Livingston, pp. 317–26.
Guilbaud, G., Peschanski, M. and Besson, J.-M. (1989) Experimental data related to nociception and pain at a supraspinal level, in P.D. Wall and R. Melzack (eds), *Textbook of Pain* (second edition), Edinburgh: Churchill Livingston, pp. 141–53.
Guillemin, F., Briancon, S. and Pourel, J. (1992) Functional disability in rheumatoid arthritis: two different models in early and established disease, *Journal of Rheumatology* 19: 366–9.
Haan, N. (1977) *Coping and defending: processes of self-environment organisation*. New York: Academic Press.
Hall, J.A., Roter, D.L. and Rand, C.S. (1981) Communication of affect between patient and physician, *Journal of Health and Social Behavior* 22: 18–30.
Harris, E. (1990) Rheumatoid arthritis: pathophysiology and implications for therapy, *New England Journal of Medicine* 322: 1277–89.
Harvey, R., Doyle, E. and Ellis, K. (1974) Major changes made by the Criteria Committee of the New York Heart Association, *Circulation* 49: 390–1.
Haug, M.R. and Ory, M.G. (1987) Issues in elderly patient–provider interactions, *Research on Aging* 9: 3–44.
Hawley, D.J. and Wolfe, F. (1988) Anxiety and depression in patients with rheumatoid arthritis: a prospective study of 400 patients, *Journal of Rheumatology* 15 (6): 932.
— (1993) Depression is not more common in rheumatoid arthritis: a 10-year longitudinal study of 6,153 patients with rheumatic disease, *The Journal of Rheumatology* 20 (12): 2025–31.
Heitzmann, C. and Kaplan, R.M. (1988) Assessment of methods for measuring social support, *Health Psychology* 7: 75–109.
Helewa, A., Goldsmith, C. and Lee, P. (1991) Effects of occupational therapy home service on patients with rheumatoid arthritis, *Lancet* 337: 1453–6.
Helewa, A., Goldsmith, C. and Smythe, H. (1982) Independent measurement of functional capacity in rheumatoid arthritis, *Journal of Epidemiology* 9: 794–7.

Heller, K., Swindle, R.W. Jr. and Dusenbury, L. (1986) Component social support processes: comments and integration, *Journal of Consulting and Clinical Psychology* 54: 466–70.

Helliwell, P.S. (1993) Joint stiffness, in V. Wright and E. Radin (eds) *Mechanics of Human Joints*: Marcel Dekker.

Helliwell, P.S. and Wright, V. (1991) Stiffness – a useful symptom but an elusive quality, *Proceedings of the Royal Society*, 95–8.

Henderson, L.J. (1935) Physician and patient as a social system, *New England Journal of Medicine* 212: 819–23.

Henderson, S., Duncan-Jones, P., Byrne, D. and Scott, R. (1980) Measuring social relationships: the Interview Schedule for Social Interaction, *Psychological Medicine* 10: 723–34.

Herzlich, C. and Pierret, J. (1985) Illness: from causes to meaning, in C. Currer and J. Pierret (eds), *Concepts of Health, Illness, and Disease: A Comparative Perspective*, Leamington Spa: Berg.

Hinrichsen, G.A., Revenson, T.A., Shinn, M. (1985) Does self-help help? An empirical investigation of scoliosis peer support groups, *Journal of Social Issues* 41: 65–87.

Hochberg, M.C., Chang, R.W., Dwosh, I., Lindsey, S., Pincus, T. and Wolfe, F. (1992) The American College of Rheumatology 1991 revised criteria for the classification of global status in rheumatoid arthritis, *Arthritis and Rheumatism* 35 (5): 418–502.

Holbrook, T., Wingard, D. and Barrett-Connor, E. (1990) Self-reported arthritis among men and women in an adult community, *Journal of Community Health* 15: 195–208.

Hopkins, A. (ed.) (1992) *Measures of the Quality of Life*, London: Royal College of Physicians.

House, J.S., and Kahn, R.L. (1985) Measures and concepts of social support, in S. Cohen & S.L. Syme (eds), *Social Support and Health*, New York: Academic Press, pp. 83–108.

Hovell, M.F. & Black, D.R. (1989) Minimal interventions and arthritis treatment: implications for patient and physician compliance, *Arthritis Care and Research* 2: S65–70.

Huskisson, E.C. (1983) Visual analogue scales, in R. Melzack (ed), *Pain measurement and assessment*, New York: Raven Press, pp. 33–7.

Huskisson, E.C. and Hart, D.F. (1978) *Joint Diseases: All the Arthropathies*, third edition, Bristol: J. Wright.

Inoue, K., Shichikawa, K., Nishioka, J., Hirota, S. (1987) Older age onset rheumatoid arthritis with or without osteoarthritis, *Annals of Rheumatic Diseases* 46: 908–11.

Jacob, D.L., Robinson, H. and Masi, A.T. (1972) A controlled home interview study of factors associated with early rheumatoid arthritis, *American Journal of Public Health* 62: 1532–37.

Jacobson, D.E. (1986) Types and timing of social support, *Journal of Health and Social Behavior*, 27: 250–64.

Jacobson, E. (1938) *Progressive Relaxation*, Chicago: University of Chicago Press.

Jayson, M.I.V. and Dixon, A. St J. (1980) *Rheumatism and arthritis: what you should know about the problems and treatment*, London: Pan.

Jenkins, R. and Clare, A. (1985) Women and mental illness, *British Medical Journal* 291: 1521–2.

Jenkinson, C., Ziebland, S., Fitzpatrick, R., Mowat, A. and Mowat, A. (1991) Sensitivity to change of weighted and unweighted versions of two health status measures, *International Journal of Health Sciences* 2: 189–94.

Jette, A. (1980) Functional status instrument: reliability of a chronic disease evaluation instrument, *Archives of Physical Medicine & Rehabilitation* 61: 395–401.

— (1982) Improving patient cooperation with arthritis treatment regimens, *Arthritis and Rheumatism* 25: 447–53.

Johnson, C.L. & Catalano, D.J. (1983) A longitudinal study of family supports to impaired elderly, *The Gerontologist* 23: 612–18.

Joint Working Group of the British Society for Rheumatology and the Research Unit of the Royal College of Physicians (1992) Guidelines and audit measures for the specialist supervision of patients with rheumatoid arthritis, *Journal of The Royal College of Physicians of London* 26: 76–82.

Kane, R.A. (1986) Family support for elderly persons with arthritis, in R.W. Moskowitz and M.R. Haug (eds), *Arthritis and the Elderly*, New York: Springer, pp. 57–71.

Kaplan, R., Anderson, J. and Ganiats, T. (1993) The Quality of Well-Being Scale: rationale for a single quality of life index, in S. Walker and R. Rosser (eds), *Quality of Life Assessment: Key Issues in the 1990s*, Dordrecht: Kluwer, pp. 65–94.

Kaplan, R.M., Coons, S.J. and Anderson, J.P. (1992) Quality of life and policy analysis in arthritis, *Arthritis Care and Research* 5: 173–83.

Kaplan, R.M., Sallis, J.F. and Patterson, T.L. (1993) *Health and Human Behavior*, New York: McGraw-Hill.

Kaplan, R.M. and Toshima, M.T. (1990) The functional effects of social relationships on chronic illnesses and disability, in B.R. Sarason, I.G. Sarason, and G.R. Pierce (eds), *Social Support: An Interactional View,* New York: John Wiley & Sons, pp. 427–53.

Kaplan, S.H., Greenfield, S. and Ware, J.E. (1989) Impact of the doctor–patient relationship on the outcomes of chronic disease, in M. Stewart and D. Roter (eds), *Communicating with Medical Patients*, Newbury Park, CA: Sage, pp. 228–45.

Karnofsky, D. and Burchenal, J. (1949) The clinical evaluation of chemotherapeutic agents in cancer, in C. McLeod (ed.), *Evaluation of Chemotherapeutic Agents,* New York: Columbia University Press, pp. 191–205.

Kazis, L., Anderson, J. and Meenan, R. (1990) Health status as a predictor of mortality in rheumatoid arthritis: a five year study, *Journal of Rheumatology* 17: 609–13.

Kazis, L., Callahan, L., Meenan, R. and Pincus, T. (1990) Health status reports in the care of patients with rheumatoid arthritis, *Journal of Clinical Epidemiology* 43: 1243–53.

Kazis, L.E., Meenan, R.F. and Anderson, J.J. (1983) Pain in the rheumatic diseases: investigation of a key healthstatus component, *Arthritis and Rheumatism* 26(8): 1017–22.

Keefe, F.J. and Block, A.R. (1982) Development of an observation method for assessing pain behaviour in chronic low back pain patients, *Behaviour Therapy* 13: 363–75.

Keefe, F.J., Brown, G.K. *et al.* (1989) Coping with rheumatoid arthritis pain: catastrophising as a maladaptive strategy, 37: 51–6.

Keefe, F.J. and van Hoorn, J. (1993) Cognitive behavioural treatment of rheumatoid arthritis pain, *Arthritis Care and Research* 6(4): 213–22.

Keeler, E.B., Solomon, D.H., Beck, J.C., Mendenhall, R.C. and Kane, R.L. (1982) Effect of patient age on duration of medical encounters with physicians, *Medical Care* 20: 1101–8.

Kelley, W.N., Harris, E.D., Ruddy, S. and Sledge, C.B. (1993) *Textbook of Rheumatology*, fourth edition, Philadelphia: W.D. Saunders.

Kelly, M.P. (1986) The subjective experience of chronic disease: some implications for the management of ulcerative colitis, *Journal of Chronic Diseases* 39: 653–66.

Kennedy, S., Kiecolt-Glaser, J.K. and Glaser, R. (1991) Social support, stress, and the immune system, in B.R. Sarason, I.G. Sarason and G.R. Pierce (eds), *Social support: an interactional view*, New York: John Wiley & Sons, pp. 253–66.

Kessler, R.C. and McLeod, J.D. (1985) Social support and mental health in community samples, in S. Cohen and S.L. Syme (eds), *Social Support and Health,* New York: Academic Press, pp. 219–40.

King, S.H. and Cobb, S. (1958) Psychosocial factors in the epidemiology of arthritis, *Journal of Chronic Diseases* 7: 466–75.

Kleinman, A. (1988) *The Illness Narratives*, New York: Basic Books.

Klipple, G. and Cecere, F. (1989) Rheumatoid arthritis and pregnancy, *Rheumatic Diseases Clinics of North America* 15: 213–39.

Kohlman, C.W. (1993) Rigid and flexible modes of coping: related to coping style, 6: 107–23.

Kronenfeld, J. and Wasner, C. (1982) The use of unorthodox therapies and marginal practitioners, *Social Science and Medicine* 16: 1119–25.

Kvitek, S.D.B., Shaver, B.J., Blood, H. and Shepard, K.F. (1986) Age bias: physical therapists and older patients, *Journal of Gerontology* 41: 706–9.

Landrine, H. and E. Klonoff (1992) Culture and health-related schemas: a review and proposal for interdisciplinary interaction, *Health Psychology*, 11: 267–76.

Lane, C. and Hobfoll, S.E. (1992) How loss affects anger and alienates potential supporters, *Journal of Consulting and Clinical Psychology* 60: 935–42.

Langley, G.B. and Sheppard, H. (1985) The visual analogue scale: its use in pain measurement, *Rheumatology International* 5: 145–8.

Lanza, A.F. and Revenson, T.A. (1993) Social support interventions for rheumatoid arthritis patients: the cart before the horse? *Health Education Quarterly* 20: 97–117.

—— (1994) Illness intrusion and psychological adjustment to rheumatic disease: the importance of social roles. Unpublished manuscript. The Graduate School & University Centre, City University of New York.

Lanza, A.F., Revenson, T.A. and Cameron, A.E. (1995) Perceptions of helpful and unhelpful support among married people with rheumatic disease, in press.

Lau, E., Symmons, D., Bankhead, C., *et al.* (1993) Low prevalence of rheumatoid arthritis in the urbanized Chinese of Hong Kong, *Journal of Rheumatology* 20: 1133–7.

Lawrence, J.S. (1970) Rheumatoid arthritis – nature or nurture? *Annals of the Rheumatic Diseases*, 29: 357–9.

Lazarus, R.S. (1993) Coping theory and research: past, present, and future, *Psychosomatic Medicine* 55: 234–47.

Lazarus, R. and Folkman, S. (1984) *Appraisal and Coping*, New York: Springer.

Lee, P. and Tan, L.J.P. (1979) Drug compliance in outpatients with rheumatoid arthritis, *Australian New Zealand Journal of Medicine* 9: 274–7.

Leigh, P. and Fries, J. (1991) Mortality predictors among 263 patients with rheumatoid arthritis, *Journal of Rheumatology* 18: 1307–12.

—— (1992) Predictors of disability in a longitudinal sample of patients with rheumatoid arthritis, *Annals of the Rheumatic Diseases* 51: 581–7.

Leserman, J. (1981) *Men and Women in Medical School*, New York: Praeger.

Leventhal, H., Nerenz, D.R. and Steele, D.J. (1984) Illness representations and coping with health threats, in A. Baum, S.E. Taylor and J.E. Singer (eds), *Handbook of Psychology and Health (volume IV): Social psychological aspects of health*, Hillsdale, New Jersey: Laurence Erblaum.

Liang, M.H. (1989) Compliance and quality of life: confessions of a difficult patient, *Arthritis Care and Research* 2: S71–4.

Liang, M.H., Cullen, K. and Larson, M. (1982) In search of the perfect mousetrap (health status or quality of life instrument), *Journal of Rheumatology* 9 (5): 775.

Liang, M.H., Larson, M., Cullen, K. and Schwartz, J. (1985) Comparative measurement efficiency and sensitivity of health status instruments for arthritis research, *Arthritis and Rheumatism* 28: 542–7.

Liang, M.H., Logigian, M.A. and Sledge, C.B. (1992) *Rehabilitation of early rheumatoid arthritis*, Boston: Little Brown & Co.

Liang, M.H., Phillips, E.E., Scamina, M.D. *et al.* (1981) Evaluation of a pilot programme for rheumatic disability in an urban community, *Arthritis and Rheumatism* 24: 937–43.

Liang, M.H., Schurman, D.J. and Fries, J. (1978) A patient-administered questionnaire for arthritis assessment, *Clinics of Orthopaedic Related Research* 131: 123–9.

Linn, M., Linn, B. and Stein, S. (1982) Beliefs about the causes of cancer in cancer patients, *Social Science and Medicine* 16: 835–9.

Linton, S.J. (1985) The relationship between activity and chronic back pain, *Pain* 24: 289–94.

Linton, S.J., Hellsing, A.L. and Anderson, D. (1993) A controlled study of the effects of an early intervention on acute musculoskeletal pain problems, *Pain* 54: 353–9.

Locker, D. (1981) *Symptoms and Illness: The Cognitive Organization of Disorder*, London: Tavistock.
— (1983) *Disability and Disadvantage: The Consequences of Chronic Illness*, London: Tavistock.
— (1989) Coping with disability and handicap, in D. Patrick and H. Peach (eds), *Disablement in the community*, Oxford: Oxford University Press, pp. 176–96.
Long, B.C. and Sangster, J.L. (1993) Dispositional optimism/pessimism and coping strategies: predictors of psychosocial adjustment of rheumatoid and osteoarthritis patients, *Journal of Applied Social Psychology* 23 (13): 1069–91.
Lorber, J. (1979) Good patients and problem patients: conformity and deviance in a general hospital, in E.G. Jaco (ed.), *Patients, physicians, and illness*, New York: Free Press, pp. 202–17.
— (1987) Mothers or MDs? Women physicians and the doctor–patient relationship, in L. Richardson and V. Taylor (eds), *Feminist frontiers II: Rethinking sex, gender and society*, New York: Random House, pp. 320–6.
Lorig, K., Chastain, R.L., Ung, E., Shoor, S. and Holman, N.R. (1989) Development and evaluation of a scale to measure perceived self-efficacy in people with arthritis, *Arthritis and Rheumatism* 32 (1): pp. 37–44.
Lorig, K.R., Cox, T., Cuevas, Y. and Britton, M.C. (1984) Converging and diverging beliefs about arthritis: Caucasian patients, Spanish speaking patients, and physicians, *Journal of Rheumatology* 11: 76–9.
Lorig, K. and Holman, H.R. (1989) Long term outcomes of an arthritis self-management study: the effects of reinforcement efforts, *Social Science and Medicine* 29 (2): 221–4.
Lorig, K., Konkol, L. and Gonzalez, V. (1987) Arthritis patient education: a review of the literature, *Patient Education and Counselling*, 10: 207–52.
Lorig, K., Mazonson, P. and Holman, H. (1993) Evidence suggesting that health education for self-management in patients with chronic arthritis has sustained health benefits while reducing healthcare costs, *Arthritis and Rheumatism* 34 (4): 439–46.
Lyle, W.H. (1984) Rheumatoid arthritis and social class (letter), *British Journal of Rheumatology* 23: 309.
McCrainie, E.W., Horowitz, A. and Martin, R.M. (1978) Alleged sex-role stereotyping in the assessment of women's physical complaints: a study of general practitioners, *Social Science and Medicine* 12: 111–16.
McDaniel, L.K., Anderson, K.O., Bradley, L.A., Young, L.D., Turner, R.A. and Keefe, F.J. (1986) Development of an observation method for assessing pain behaviour in rheumatoid arthritis, *Pain*, 24: 165–84.
McEwen, J. (1993) The Nottingham Health Profile, in S. Walker and R. Rosser (eds), *Quality of Life Assessment: Key Issues in the 1990s*, Dordrecht: Kluwer, pp. 111–30.
McFarlane, A., Brooks, P. (1988) An analysis of the relationship between psychological morbidity and disease activity in rheumatoid arthritis, *Journal of Rheumatology* 15: 926–31.

McGowan, P. (1988) Arthritis men's group. *Arthritis Care and Research* 1: 53–56.

McGrath, E. and Zimet, C.W. (1977) Female and male medical students: differences in specialty choice selection and personality, *Journal of Medical Education* 52: 293–300.

MacGregor, A.J., Riste, L.K., Hazes, J.M. *et al.* (1994) Low prevalence of rheumatoid arthritis in black-Caribbeans compared with whites in inner city Manchester, *Annals of the Rheumatic Diseases* 53: 293–7.

Mackenzie, R., Charlson, M., DiGiola, D. and Kelly, K. (1986) Can the Sickness Impact Profile measure change? An example of scale assessment, *Journal of Chronic Diseases* 39: 429–38.

McQuay, H. (1990) Assessment of pain and effectiveness of treatment in A. Hopkins and D. Costain (eds) *Measuring the Outcomes of Medical Care*, London: Royal College of Physicians, 43–57.

McQuay, H.J. (1991) Opioid clinical pharmacology and routes of administration, *British Medical Bulletin*, 47: 703–17.

Maddison, P.J., Isenberg, D.A., Woo, P. *et al.* (1993) *Oxford Textbook of Rheumatology*, Oxford: Oxford University Press.

Majerovitz, S.D., Revenson, T.A. (1992) Stability and change in social networks and social support among individuals facing a chronic stressor. Unpublished manuscript.

Manne, S. and Zautra, A. (1989) Spouse criticism and support: their association with coping and psychological adjustment among women with rheumatoid arthritis, *Journal of Personality and Social Psychology*, 56: 608–17.

— (1990) Couples coping with chronic illness: women with rheumatoid arthritis and their healthy husbands, *Journal of Behavioral Medicine* 13 (4): 327–43.

— (1992) Coping with arthritis, *Arthritis and Rheumatism* 35 (11): 1273–80.

Martin, J., Meltzer, H. and Elliott, D. (1988) *The Prevalence of Disability Among Adults*, London: HMSO.

Martin, S.C., Arnold, R.M. and Parker, R.M. (1988) Gender and medical socialization, *Journal of Health and Social Behavior* 29: 333–43.

Mason, J., Anderson, J. and Meenan, R. (1988) A model of health status for rheumatoid arthritis, *Arthritis and Rheumatism* 31: 714–20.

Mason, J.H., Anderson, J.J., Meenan, R.F., Haralson, K.M., Lewis-Stevens, D. and Kaine, J.L. (1992) The Rapid Assessment of Disease Activity in Rheumatology (RADAR) Questionnaire – validity and sensitivity to change of a patient self report measure of joint count and clinical status, *Arthritis and Rheumatism* 35 (2): 156–62.

Mason, J.H., Weener, J.L., Gertman, P.M. and Meenan, R.F. (1983) Health status in chronic disease: a comparative study of rheumatoid arthritis, *Journal of Rheumatology* 10: 763–8.

Maton, K.I. (1988) Social support, organizational characteristics, psychological well-being, and group appraisal in three self-help group populations, *American Journal of Community Psychology* 16: 53–77.

Mechanic, D. (1976) Sex, illness behavior and the use of the health services, *Journal of Human Stress* 2: 29–40.
Medsger, A.R. and Robinson, H. (1972) A comparative study of divorce in rheumatoid arthritis and other rheumatic diseases, *Journal of Chronic Disease* 25: 269–75.
Meenan, R.F. (1982) The AIMS approach to health status measurement: conceptual backgrounds and measurement properties, *Journal of Rheumatology* 9: 785–9.
— (1991) Rheumatology manpower – the US perspective (editorial), *British Journal of Rheumatology* 30: 81.
Meenan, R., Anderson, J., Kazis, L., Egger, M., Altz-Smith, M., Samuelson, C., Wilkens, R., Solsky, M., Hayes, S., Blocka, K., Weinstein, A., Guttadauria, M., Kaplan, S. and Klippel J. (1984) Outcome assessment in clinical trials: evidence for the sensitivity of a health status measure, *Arthritis and Rheumatism* 27: 1433–52.
Meenan, R.F., Gertman, P.M., and Mason, J.H. (1980) Measuring health status in arthritis: the Arthritis Impact Measurement Scales, *Arthritis and Rheumatism* 23(2): 146–52.
Meenan, R.F., Gertman, P.M., Mason, J.H. and Dunaif, R. (1982) The Arthritis Impact Measurement Scales: further investigations of a measure, *Arthritis and Rheumatism* 25(9): 1048–53.
Meenan, R., Mason, J., Anderson, J., Guccione, A. and Kazis, L. (1992) The content and properties of a revised and expanded arthritis impact measurement scales health status questionnaire, *Arthritis and Rheumatism* 35: 1–10.
Meenan, R.F., Yelin, E.H. *et al.* (1981) The impact of chronic disease: a sociomedical profile of rheumatoid arthritis 24(3): 544–9.
Melamed, B.G. and Brenner, G.F. (1989) Social support and chronic medical stress: an interaction-based approach, *Journal of Social and Clinical Psychology* 9: 104–17.
Melzack, R. (1975) The McGill Pain Questionnaire – major properties and scoring methods, *Pain* 1: 277–99.
— (1987) The short-form McGill Pain Questionnaire, *Pain* 30: 191–7.
Melzack, R. and Dennis, S.G. (1978) Neurophysiological foundations of pain, in R.A. Sternbach (ed.) *The Psychology of Pain*, New York: Raven Press: 1–26.
Melzack, R. and Wall, P.D. (1965) The gate control theory of pain, *Science N.Y.* 150: 971–9.
— (1982) *The Challenge of Pain*, second edition (third edition 1988), Harmondsworth: Penguin.
Miall, W.E., Caplan, A., Cochrane, A.L. *et al.* (1953) An epidemiological study of rheumatoid arthritis associated with characteristic chest X-ray appearances in coal workers, *British Medical Journal* 4: 1231–6.
Miles, A. (1991) *Women, health and medicine*, Milton Keynes, England: Open University Press.
Mitchell, J., Burkhauser, R. and Pincus, T. (1988) The importance of age, education and comorbidity in the substantial earnings losses of individuals with symmetric polyarthritis, *Arthritis and Rheumatism* 31: 348–57.

Monks, R. and Taenzer, P. (1983) A comprehensive pain questionnaire, in R. Melzack (ed.), *Pain measurement and assessment*, New York: Raven Press, pp. 233–7.

Moon, M.H., Moon, B.A.M. and Black, W.A.M. (1976) Compliancy in splint-wearing behaviour of patients with rheumatoid arthritis, *New Zealand Medical Journal* 83: 360–5.

Morgan, M. (1989) Social ties, support and well-being, in D. Patrick and H. Peach (eds), *Disablement in the Community*, Oxford: Oxford University Press.

Morgan, M., Patrick, D.L. and Charlton, J.R. (1984) Social networks and psychosocial support among disabled people, *Social Science and Medicine* 19: 489–97.

Murphy, S., Creed, F. *et al.* (1988) Psychiatric disorder and illness behaviour in rheumatoid arthritis, *British Journal of Rheumatology* 27: 357–63.

Murray, M. (1990) Lay representations of illness, in P. Bennett, J. Weinman and P. Spurgeone (eds), *Current Developments in Health Psychology*, London: Harwood Academic Publishers, pp. 63–92.

Nehemkis, A.M., Keenan, M.A., Person, D. and Prete, P.E. (1985) The nature of arthritis pain, *British Journal of Rheumatology* 24: 53–60.

Nelson, E., Landgraf, J., Hays, R., Wasson, J. and Kirk, J. (1990) The functional status of patients. How can it be measured in physicians' offices? *Medical Care* 28: 1111–26.

Neuberger, G., Smith, K.V., Black, S.O. and Hassanein, R. (1993) Promoting self care in clients with arthritis, *Arthritis Care and Research* 6(3): 141–8.

Newman, S. (1990) Coping with chronic illness, *Current Developments in Health Psychology*. London: Harwood, pp. 159–75.

—— (1993) Coping with rheumatoid arthritis, *Annals of the Rheumatic Diseases* 53: 553–4.

Newman, S. and Durrance, P. (1994) *The Context of Cognitions and Expectations*. Internat Association of Applied Psychology Conference, Madrid.

Newman, S.P., Fitzpatrick, R. *et al.* (1989) The origins of depressed mood in rheumatoid arthritis, *Journal of Rheumatology* 16: 740–4.

—— (1990) Patterns of coping in rheumatoid arthritis, *Psychology and Health* 4: 187–200.

Newman, S. and Revenson, T.A. (1993) Coping with rheumatoid arthritis, in S. Newman and M. Shipley (eds) *Psychological Aspects of Rheumatic Disease. Baillière's Clinical Rheumatology*, 7(2): 259–80. London: Baillière Tindall.

Nuttbrock, L. and Kosberg, J.I. (1980) Images of the physician and help-seeking behavior of the elderly: a multivariate assessment, *Journal of Gerontology* 35: 241–8.

Oakes, T.W., Ward, J.R., Gray, R.M., Klauber, M.R. and Moody, P.M. (1970) Family expectations and arthritis patient compliance to a hand resting splint regimen, *Journal of Chronic Diseases* 22: 757–64.

Oakley, A. (1985) *The Sociology of Housework*, second edition, Oxford: Basil Blackwell.

O'Boyle, C., McGee, H., Hickey, A., O'Malley, K. and Joyce, C. (1992) Individual quality of life in patients undergoing hip replacement, *Lancet* 339: 1088–91.

O'Leary, A. (1985) Self-efficacy and health, *Behaviour Research and Therapy* 23(4): 437–51.

O'Reilly, P. (1988) Methodological issues in social support and social network research, *Social Science and Medicine* 26: 863–73.

Papageorgiou, A.C. (1994) Fatigue in rheumatoid arthritis. Unpublished M.Sc dissertation, Faculty of Medicine, University of Manchester.

Papageorgiou, A.C., and Badley, E.M. (1989) The quality of pain in arthritis: the words patients use to describe overall pain and pain in individual joints at rest and on movement, *Journal of Rheumatology* 16(1): 106.

Parker, J.D. and Endler, N.S. (1992) Coping with coping assessment: a critical review, *European Journal of Personality* 6: 321–44.

Parker, J., Frank, R., Beck, N., Finan, M., Walker, S., Hewett, J.E., Broster, C., Smarr, K., Smith, E. and Kay, D. (1988) Pain in rheumatoid arthritis: relationship to demographic medical and psychological factors, *Journal of Rheumatology* 15(3): 433.

Parker, J.C., Iverson, G.L., Smarr, K.L. and Stucky-Ropp, R.C. (1993) Cognitive-behavioural approaches to pain management in rheumatoid arthritis, *Arthritis Care and Research* 6(4): 207–12.

Parker, J., McRae, C. *et al.* (1988) Coping strategies in rheumatoid arthritis, 15(9): 1376–83.

Parker, J.C., Smarr, K.L., Angelone, E.O., Mothersead, P.K., Lee, B.S., Walker, S.E., Bridges, A.J. and Caldwell, C.W. (1992) Psychological factors, immunologic activation and disease activity in rheumatoid arthritis, *Arthritis Care and Research* 5(4): 196–201.

Partridge, R.E.H. and Duthie, J.J.R. (1968) Rheumatism in dockers and civil servants: a comparison of heavy manual and sedentary workers, *Annals of the Rheumatic Diseases* 27: 559–69.

Pathria, M., Bjorkengren, A., Jacob, J. *et al.* (1988) Rheumatoid arthritis: similarity of radiographic abnormalities in men and women, *Radiology* 167: 793–5.

Patrick, D., Morgan, M. and Charlton, J. (1986) Psychosocial support and change in the health status of physically disabled people, *Social Science and Medicine* 22: 1347–54.

Patrick, D. and Peach, H. (eds) (1989) *Disablement in the community*, Oxford: Oxford University Press.

Pearlin, L.I. (1989) Sociological study of stress, *Journal of Health and Social Behavior* 30: 241–56.

Pearlin, L. and Schooler, C. (1978) The structure of coping, *Journal of Health and Social Behaviour* 19: 2–21.

Peck, J.R., Smith, W. *et al.* (1989) Disability and depression in rheumatoid arthritis: a multi-trait, multi-method investigation, *Arthritis and Rheumatism* 32 (9): 1100–6.

Pennebaker, J.W. (1982) *The Psychology of Physical Symptoms*, New York: Springer Verlag.

Pilgrim, D. and Rogers, A. (1983) *A sociology of mental health and illness*, Buckingham: Open University Press.

Pill, R. and Stott, N. (1982) Concepts of illness causation and responsibility: some preliminary data from a sample of working class mothers, *Social Science and Medicine* 16: 43–52.

Pinals, R. (1987) Survival in rheumatoid arthritis, *Arthritis and Rheumatism* 30: 473–5.

Pincus, T. and Callahan, L. (1985) Formal education as a marker for increased mortality and morbidity in rheumatoid arthritis, *Journal of Chronic Diseases* 38: 973–84.

—— (1986) Taking mortality in rheumatoid arthritis seriously – predictive markers, socioeconomic status, and co-morbidity, *Journal of Rheumatology* 13: 841–5.

—— (1993a) The side effects of rheumatoid arthritis: joint destruction, disability and early mortality, *British Journal of Rheumatology* 32 (Supp. 1): 28–37.

—— (1993b) What is the natural history of rheumatoid arthritis? *Rheumatic Disease Clinics of North America* 19: 123–51.

Pincus, T., Callahan, L.F. *et al.* (1986) Elevated MMPI scores for hypochondriasis, depression and hysteria in patients with rheumatoid arthritis reflects disease rather than psychosocial status, *Arthritis and Rheumatism* 29: 1456–66.

Pincus, T., Summey, J., Soraci, S. *et al.* (1983) Assessment of patient satisfaction in activities of daily living using a modified Stanford Health Assessment Questionnaire, *Arthritis and Rheumatism* 26: 1346–53.

Popay, J. (1991) My health is alright but I'm tired all the time: women's experiences of ill-health, in H. Roberts (ed.), *Women's Health Matters*, London: Routledge, pp. 99–120.

Popay, J. and Williams, G.H. (eds) (1994) *Researching the People's Health*, London: Routledge.

Porter, D. and Sturrock, R. (1993) Medical management of rheumatoid arthritis, *British Medical Journal* 307: 425–8.

Potts, M.K., Mazzuca, S.A., and Brandt, K.D. (1986) View of patients and physicians regarding the importance of various aspects of arthritis treatment: correlations with health status and patient satisfaction, *Patient Education and Counseling* 8: 124–5.

Potts, M.K., Weinberger, M. and Brandt, K.D. (1984) Views of patients and providers regarding the importance of various aspects of an arthritis treatment program, *Journal of Rheumatology* 11: 71–5.

Price, J.H., Hillman, K.S., Toralt, M.E. and Newell, S. (1983) The public's perception and misperception of arthritis, *Arthritis and Rheumatism* 26 (8): 1023–8.

Prior, P. and Symmons, D.P.M. (1984) Rheumatoid arthritis and social class (reply to Lyle), *British Journal of Rheumatology* 23: 310.

Prior, P., Symmons, D.P.M., Scott, D.L., *et al.* (1984) Cause of death in rheumatoid arthritis, *British Journal of Rheumatology* 23: 92–9.

Pritchard, M.L. (1989) *Psychological aspects of rheumatoid arthritis*, New York: Springer-Verlag.

Probstfield, J.L. (1989) Adherence and its management in clinical trials: implications for arthritis treatment trials, *Arthritis Care and Research* 2: S48–57.

Radley, A. (1989) Style, discourse and constraint in adjustment of chronic illness, *Sociology of Health and Illness* 11: 230–52.

— (ed) (1993) *Worlds of illness: biographical and cultural perspectives on health and disease*, London: Routledge.

Radojevic, V., Nicassio, P.M. and Weisman, M.H. (1992) Behavioral intervention with and without family support for rheumatoid arthritis, *Behavior Therapy* 23: 13–30.

Randlich, A. (1993) Neural substrates of pain and analgesia, *Arthritis Care and Research* 6(4): 171–7.

Rapoff, M.A. (1989) Compliance with treatment regimens for pediatric rheumatic diseases, *Arthritis Care and Research* 2: S40–7.

Rasker, J. and Cosh, J. (1992) Long term effects of treating RA, in D. Scott (ed.) *Baillière's Clinical Rheumatology: the Course and Outcome of Rheumatoid Arthritis*, London, Baillière Tindall, pp. 141–60.

Ray, C., Lindop, J. and Gibson, S. (1982) The concept of coping, *Psychological Medicine* 12: 385–95.

Reisine, S. (1993) Marital status and social support in Rheumatoid Arthritis, *Arthritis and Rheumatism* 36(5): 589–92.

Reisine, S. and Fifield, J. (1992) Expanding the definition of disability: implications for planning, policy and research, *Milbank Quarterly* 70: 491–508.

Reisine, S., Goodenow, C. and Grady, K. (1987) The impact of rheumatoid arthritis on the homemaker, *Social Science and Medicine* 25: 89–96.

Revenson, T.A. (1989) Compassionate stereotyping of elderly patients by physicians, *Psychology and Aging* 4: 230–4.

— (1990) All other things are *not* equal: An ecological perspective on the relation between personality and disease, in H.S. Friedman (ed), *Personality and Disease*, New York: John Wiley, pp. 65–94.

— (1993) The role of social support with rheumatic disease, in S. Newman and M. Shipley (eds), *Psychological aspects of rheumatic disease. Baillière's clinical rheumatology*, 7(2): 377–96. London: Baillière Tindal.

— (1994) Social support and marital coping with chronic illness, *Annals of Behavioral Medicine* 16(2): 122–30.

Revenson, T.A. and Cameron, A. (1992) *Coping processes amongst married couples with rheumatic disease*. Paper presented at the American Psychological Association, Washington, DC.

Revenson, T.A., Cameron, A.E. and Gibosky, A. (1992, November) Age and gender stereotyping by physicians: is there a double standard? in M.G. Ory (Chair), *Current research on the physician–older patient relationship*. Symposium presented at the Annual Meeting of the Gerontological Society of America, Washington, DC.

Revenson, T.A. and Felton, B.J. (1989) Disability and coping as predictors of psychological adjustment to rheumatoid arthritis.

Revenson, T.A. and Majerovitz, S.D. (1990) Spouses' support provision to chronically ill patients, *Journal of Social and Personal Relationships* 7: 575–86.

— (1991) The effects of illness on the spouse: social resources as stress buffers, *Arthritis Care and Research* 4: 63–72.

Revenson, T.A., Schiaffino, K.M., Majerovitz, S.D. and Gibofsky, A. (1991) Social support as a double-edged sword: the relation of positive and problematic support to depression among rheumatoid arthritis patients, *Social Science and Medicine* 33: 801–13.

Revenson, T.A., Wollman, C.A. and Felton, B.J. (1983) Social supports as stress buffers for adult cancer patients, *Psychosomatic Medicine* 45: 321–30.

Rhind, V.M., Bird, H.A. and Wright, V. (1980) Comparison of clinical assessments of disease activity in rheumatoid arthritis, *Annals of the Rheumatic Diseases* 39: 135–7.

Rigby, A.S. and Wood, P.H. (1990) A review of assignment criteria for rheumatoid arthritis, *Scandinavian Journal of Rheumatology* 19: 27–41.

Rimon, R. (1974) Depression in rheumatoid arthritis: prevalence by self-report questionnaire and recognition by nonpsychiatric physicians, *Annals of Clinical Research* 6: 171–5.

Robins, H.S. and Walters, K. (1971) Return to work after treatment of rheumatoid arthritis, *Canadian Medical Association Journal* 105: 166–9.

Robins, N., Hlezer, J., Croughan, J. and Ratcliff, K. (1981) National Institute of Mental Health Diagnostic Interview Schedule. Its history, characteristics and validity, *Archives of General Psychiatry* 38: 381–9.

Rodin, G., Craven, J. and Littlefield, C. (1991) *Depression in the medically ill: an integrated approach*, New York: Brunner-Mazel.

Rodin, J. and Janis, I.L. (1982) The social influence of physicians and other health care practitioners as agents of change, in H.S. Friedman and M.R. DiMatteo (eds), *Interpersonal Issues in Health Care*, New York: Academic Press, pp. 33–49.

Romano, J.M. and Turner, J.A. (1985) Chronic pain and depression: does the evidence support the relationship? *Psychological Bulletin* 97: 18–34.

Rook, K.S. (1990) Social networks as a source of social control in older adults' lives, in H. Giles, N. Coupland, J.M. Wiemann (eds), *Communication, health and the elderly*, Manchester, England: Manchester University Press, pp. 45–63.

Ropes, M.W., Bennett, G.A., Cobb, S., Jacox, R. and Jessar, R.A. (1958) Revision of diagnostic criteria for rheumatoid arthritis, *Bulletin on Rheumatic Diseases* IX (4): 175–6.

Rosenberg, M. (1965) *Society and the adolescent self image*, Princeton, NJ: Princeton University Press.

Rosenstiel, A.K. and Keefe, F.J. (1983) The use of coping strategies in chronic low back pain patients: relationship to patients' characteristics and current adjustment, *Pain* 17: 33–40.

Ross, C.K., Sinacore, Steirs, J.M. and Budiman-Mak, E. (1990) The role of expectations and preferences in health care satisfaction of patients with arthritis, *Arthritis Care and Research* 3: 92–8.

Roter, D., Lipkin, M. and Korsgaard, A. (1991) Sex differences in patients' and physicians' communication during primary care medical visits, *Medical Care* 29: 1083–93.

Rudick, R., Miller, D., Clough, J., Gragg, L. and Farmer, R. (1992) Quality of life in multiple sclerosis: comparison with inflammatory bowel disease and rheumatoid arthritis, *Archives of Neurology* 49: 1237–42.

Russell, D.W. and Cutrona, C.E. (1991) Social support, stress, and depressive symptoms among the elderly: test of a process model, *Psychology and Aging* 6: 190–201.

Rybstein-Blinchik (1979) Effects of different cognitive strategies on chronic pain experience, *Journal of Behavioral Medicine* 2: 93–101.

Sarason, S.B. (1985) *Caring and compassion in clinical practice*. San Francisco: Jossey-Bass. Training of physicians: The unintended impact of the Flexner report on medical education, pp. 38–61.

Scheier, M.F., Weintraub, J.K. *et al.* (1986) Coping with stress: divergent strategies of optimists and pessimists, *Journal of Personality and Social Psychology* 51: 1257–64.

Schiaffino, K.M., Revenson, T.A. and Gibofsky, A. (1991) Assessing the impact of self-efficacy beliefs on adaptation to rheumatoid arthritis, *Arthritis Care and Research* 4 (4): 150–7.

Schneider, J.W. and Conrad, P. (1983) *Having epilepsy: the experience and control of illness*, Philadelphia: Temple University Press.

Schulz, R. and Tompkins, C. (1990) Life events and changes in social relationships: examples, mechanisms and measurement, *Journal of Social and Clinical Psychology* 9: 69–77.

Schwarzer, R. and Leppin, A. (1989) Social support and health: a meta-analysis, *Psychology and Health* 3: 1–15.

Scott, D. and Huskisson, E. (1992) The course of rheumatoid arthritis, in D. Scott (ed.) *Baillière's Clinical Rheumatology: The Course and Outcome of Rheumatoid Arthritis*, London: Baillière Tindall, pp. 1–22.

Scott, D., Symmons, D., Coulton, B. and Popert, A. (1987) Long term outcome of treating rheumatoid arthritis: results after 20 years, *Lancet* i: 1108–11.

Scott, J.T. (ed.), (1986) *Copeman's textbook of the rheumatic diseases,* sixth edition, London: Churchill Livingstone.

Seijo, R., Gomez, H. and Friedenberg, J. (1991) Language as a communication barrier in medical care for Hispanic patients, *Hispanic Journal of Behavioral Sciences* 13: 363–76.

Sensky, T. and Catalan, J. (1992) Asking patients about their treatment, *British Medical Journal* 305: 1109–10.

Sewell, K. and Trentham, D. (1993) Pathogenesis of rheumatoid arthritis, *Lancet* 341: 2836.

Shapiro, J. (1990) Patterns of psychosocial performance in the d–p encounter: a study of family practice residents, *Social Science and Medicine* 31: 1035–41.

Sharma, U. (1992) *Complementary medicine today: practitioners and patients*, London: Routledge.

Sherrer, Y., Bloch, D., Mitchell, D., *et al.* (1986) The development of disability in rheumatoid arthritis, *Annals of Rheumatic Diseases* 29: 494–500.

Shmerling, R. and Delbanco, T. (1992) How useful is the rheumatoid factor? *Archives of Internal Medicine* 152: 2417–20.

Shumacher, S.A. and Brownell, A. (1984) Toward a theory of social support: closing conceptual gaps, *Journal of Social Issues* 40: 11–36.

Shumaker, S.A. and Hill, D.R. (1991) Gender differences in social support and physical health, *Health Psychology* 10: 102–11.

Singh, G., Fries, J., Williams, C., *et al.* (1991) Toxicity profiles of disease-modifying antirheumatic drugs in rheumatoid arthritis, *Journal of Rheumatology* 18: 188–94.

Skevington, S.M. (1979) Pain and locus of control: a social approach, in D.J. Osborne, M.M. Gruneberg and J.R. Eiser (eds) *Research in Psychology and Medicine*, Vol. 1, London: Academic Press, pp. 61–9.

— (1983) Chronic pain and depression: universal or personal helplessness? *Pain* 15: 309–17.

— (1986) Psychological aspects of pain in rheumatoid arthritis: a review, *Social Science and Medicine* 23(6): 567–75.

— (1991) Pain control and mechanisms for the measurement of pain, *Journal of Psychopharmacology* 5(4): 360–3.

— (1993) Depression and causal attributions in the early stages of a chronic painful disease: a longitudinal study of early synovitis, *Psychology and Health* 8: 51–64.

— (1994) The relationship between pain and depression: a longitudinal study of early synovitis, in G.F. Gebhart, D.L. Hammond, and T.S. Jensen (eds), *Proceedings of the 7th World Congress on Pain. Progress in Pain Research and Management*, Vol. 2, Seattle, IASP: Press, pp. 201–10.

Skevington, S.M. (1995) *Psychology of Pain,* Chichester: John Wiley and Sons.

Smith, C.A., Dobbins, C.J. and Wallston, K.A. (1991) The mediational role of perceived competence in psychological adjustment to rheumatoid arthritis, *Journal of Applied Social Psychology* 21: 1218–47.

Smith, C.A. and Wallston, K. (1993) *Validation of a multidimensional pain coping inventory*. Twenty-eighth National Scientific Meeting of the Arthritis Health Professions Association, San Antonio.

Smith, T.W., Peck, J.R., Milano, R.A. and Ward, J.R. (1988) Cognitive distortions in rheumatoid arthritis: relation to depression and disability, *Journal of Consulting and Clinical Psychology* 56 (3): 412–16.

Solomon, K. and Vickers, R. (1979) Attitudes of health workers toward old people, *Journal of the American Geriatrics Society*, 27: 186–91.

Sontag, S. (1979) The double standard of aging, in J. Williams (ed.), *Psychology of women*, New York: Academic Press, pp. 462–78.

Spector, T. (1991) The epidemiology of rheumatic diseases, *Current Opinion in Rheumatology* 3: 266–71.

Spector, T. and Hochberg, M. (1990) The protective effect of the OC pill on RA, *Journal of Clinical Epidemiology* 43: 1221–30.

Speeling, E.J. and Rose, D.N. (1985) Building an effective doctor–patient relationship: from patient satisfaction to patient participation, *Social Science and Medicine* 21(2): 115–20.

Spence, D., Feigenbaum, E., Fitzgerald, R. and Roth, J. (1968) Medical student attitudes toward the geriatric patient, *Journal of the American Geriatrics Society* 16: 976–83.

Spiegel, J., Leake, B., Spiegel, T., Paulus, H., Kane, R., Ward, N. and Ware, J. (1988) What are we measuring: an examination of self-reported functional status measures, *Arthritis and Rheumatism* 31: 721–8.

Sprangers, M., and Aaronson, N. (1992) The role of health care providers and significant others in evaluating the quality of life of patients with chronic disease: a review, *Journal of Clinical Epidemiology* 45: 743–60.

Steinbrocker, O., Traeger, C. and Batterman, R. (1949) Therapeutic criteria in rheumatoid arthritis, *Journal of American Medical Association* 140: 659–62.

Stewart, A., Greenfield, S., Hays, R., Wells, K., Rogers, W., Berry, S., McGlynn, A. and Ware, J. (1989) Functional status and well-being of patients with chronic conditions, *Journal of American Medical Association* 262: 907–13.

Stewart, D.C. and Sullivan, T.J. (1982) Illness behaviour and the sick role in chronic disease: the case of multiple sclerosis, *Social Science and Medicine* 16: 1297–1404.

Stiles, W.B., Putnam, S.M., Wolf, M.H. and James, S.A. (1979) Interaction exchange structure and patient satisfaction with medical interview, *Medical Care* 17: 667–79.

Stone, A.A., Kennedy-Moore, E. *et al.* (1992) Conceptual and methodological issues in current coping assessments. *Personal coping theory, research and applications*, Westport: Praeger.

Stone, A. and Neale, J. (1984) New measure of daily coping: development and preliminary results. *Journal of Personality and Social Psychology* 46: 892–906.

Sullivan, F., Eagers, R., Lynch, K. and Barber, J. (1987) Assessment of disability caused by rheumatic diseases in general practice. *Annals of the Rheumatic Diseases* 46: 598–600.

Sullivan, M., Ahlmen, M. and Bjelle, A. (1990) Health status assessment in rheumatoid arthritis. 1. Further work on the validity of the Sickness Impact Profile, *Journal of Rheumatology* 17: 439–47.

Symmons, D.P.M., Jones, S. and Hothersall, T.E. (1991) Rheumatology manpower in the 1990s', *British Journal of Rheumatology* 30: 119–22.

Szasz, T.S. & Hollender, M.H. (1956) The basic models of the doctor–patient relationship, *Archives of Internal Medicine* 97: 585–92.

Tack, B. (1990) Fatigue in rheumatoid arthritis, *Arthritis Care and Research* 3: 65–70.

Tait, R.C., Chibnall, J.T. and Krause, S. (1990) The Pain Disability Index: psychometric properties, *Pain* 40: 171–82.

Tardy, C.H. (1985) Social support measurement, *American Journal of Community Psychology* 13: 187–202.

Taylor, S.E. (1982) Hospital patient behavior: reactance, helplessness and control, in H.S. Friedman & M.R. DiMatteo (eds), *Interpersonal issues in health care*, New York: Academic Press, pp. 209–32.

Teasdale, J.D. (1983) Negative thinking in depression: cause, effect or reciprocal relationship, *Advances in Behaviour Research and Therapy* 5: 3–25.

Teasdale, J.D. (1985) Psychological treatments for depression – how do they work? *Behaviour Research and Therapy* 23(1) 157–65.

Tennen, H., Affleck, G., Urrows, S., Higgins, P. and Mendola, R. (1992) Perceiving control, construing benefits and daily processes in rheumatoid arthritis, *Canadian Journal of Behavioural Science* 24: 186–203.

Tennen, H. and Herzberger, S. (1985) Ways of Coping Scale, *Test Critiques*. Kansas City: Test Corporation of America, pp. 686–97.

Thoits, P.A. (1982) Conceptual, methodological, and theoretical problems in studying social support as a buffer against life stress, 23 (June): 145–59.

—(1986) Social support as coping assistance, *Journal of Consulting and Clinical Psychology* 54: 416–23.

Thompson, P. and Pegley, F. (1991) A comparison of disability measured by the Stanford Health Assessment Questionnaire Disability Scales (HAQ) in male and female rheumatoid outpatients, *British Journal of Rheumatology* 30: 298–300.

Thompson, S.C. and Sobolew-Shubin, A. (1993) Overprotective relationships: a nonsupportive side of social networks, *Basic and Applied Social Psychology* 14: 363–83.

Tousignant, M., Brosseau, R. and Tremblay, L. (1987) Sex biases in mental health scales: do women tend to report less serious symptoms and confide more than men? *Psychological Medicine* 17: 203–15.

Townsend, P., Davidson, N. and Whitehead, M. (1988) *The Black Report/The health divide*, Harmondsworth: Penguin.

Travis, C.B. (1988) *Women and health psychology*, Hillsdale, NJ: Lawrence Erlbaum Associates.

Tugwell, P., Bombardier, C., Bell, M., Bennett, K., Bensen, W., Grace, E., Hart, L. and Goldsmith, C. (1991) Current quality of life research challenges in arthritis relevant to the issue of clinical significance, *Controlled Clinical Trials* 12: 217S–25.

Tugwell, P., Bombardier, C., Buchanan, W., Goldsmith, C., Grace, E. and Bennett, K. (1990) Methotrexate in rheumatoid arthritis: impact on quality of life assessed by traditional standard-item and individualized patient preference health status questionnaires, *Archives of Internal Medicine* 150: 59–62.

Tugwell, P., Bombardier, C., Buchanan, W., Goldsmith, C., Grace, E. and Hanna, B. (1987) The MACTAR Patient Preference Disability Questionnaire: an individualized functional priority approach for assessing improvement in physical disability in clinical trials in rheumatoid arthritis, *Journal of Rheumatology* 14: 446–51.

Tversky, A. and Kahneman, D. (1974) Judgment under uncertainty: heuristics and biases, *Science* 185: 1124–31.

Turk, D.C., Meichenbaum, D. and Genest, M. (1983) *Pain and Behavioral Medicine: A Cognitive Behavioral Perspective*, New York: Guildford.

Vaillant, G.E. (1977) *Adaptation to Life*, Boston: Little Brown.

Vandenbroucke, J., Valkenburg, H., Boersma, J., *et al.* (1982) Oral contraceptives and rheumatoid arthritis: further evidence for a preventive effect, *Lancet* 2: 839–42.

Varni, J.W. (1981) Self-regulation techniques in the management of chronic arthritic pain in haemophilia, *Behaviour Therapy* 12: 185–94.

Veit, C.T. and J.E. Ware (1983) 'The structure of psychological distress and well-being in general populations, 51(5): 730–42.

Verbrugge, L.M. (1980) Sex differences in complaints and diagnoses, *Journal of Behavioral Medicine* 3: 327–55.

Verbrugge, L., Gates, D. and Ike, R. (1991) Risk factors for disability among US adults with arthritis, *Journal of Clinical Epidemiology* 44: 167–82.

Verbrugge, L.M. and Steiner, R.P. (1984) Another look at physicians' treatment of men and women with common complaints, *Sex Roles* 11: 1091–1109.

Vernon-Roberts, B. (1975) The applied anatomy of joints. In M. Mason and H.-F. Currey (eds), *An introduction to clinical rheumatology*, second edition, Bath: Pitman.

Waggoner, C.D. and Le Lieuvre, R.B. (1981) A method to increase compliance to exercise regimens in rheumatoid arthritis patients, *Journal of Behavioral Medicine* 4(2): 191–201.

Wagstaff, S., Smith, O.V. and Wood, P.H.N. (1985) Verbal pain descriptors used by patients with arthritis, *Annals of the Rheumatic Diseases* 44: 262–5.

Waitzkin, H. (1983) *The second sickness: contradictions of capitalist health care*, Glencoe: The Free Press.

Waldron, I. (1983) Sex differences in illness incidence, prognosis and mortality: issues and evidence, *Social Science and Medicine* 17: 1107–23.

Walker, S. and Rosser, R. (eds) (1993) *Quality of Life Assessment: Key Issues in the 1990s.* Dordrecht: Kluwer Academic Publishers.

Wallen, J., Waitzkin, H. and Stoeckle, J.D. (1979) Physicians' stereotypes about female health and illness: a study of patients' sex and the informative process during medical interviews, *Women and Health* 4: 135–46.

Wall, P.D. and Melzack, R. (1989) *Textbook of Pain* (2nd edn), Edinburgh: Churchill Livingstone.

Waller, K. (1988) Women doctors for women patients? *British Journal of Medical Psychology* 61: 125–35.

Wallston, B.S., Alagna, S.W., DeVellis, B.M. and DeVellis, R.F. (1983) Social support and physical health, *Health Psychology* 2: 367–91.

Wallston, K.A., Brown, G.K., Stein, M.J. and Dobbins, C.J. (1989) Comparing the short and long versions of the AIMS, *Journal of Rheumatology* 16(8): 1105.

Wallston, K.A. and DeVellis, B.M. (1991) *The Effects of Arthritis on Psychological Well-being*, St Louis, MO: Biopsychosocial Determinants of Arthritis Disability.

Ward, M.M. and Leigh, J.P. (1993) Marital status and the progression of functional disability in patients with rheumatoid arthritis, *Arthritis and Rheumatism* 36 (5): 581–8.

Ware, J., and Sherbourne, C. (1992) The MOS 36-item Short Form Health Survey (SF-36), *Medical Care* 30: 473–83.

Weinberger, M., Hiner, S. and Tierney, W. (1986) Improving functional status in arthritis: the effect of social support, *Social Science and Medicine* 23: 899–904.

Weinberger, M., Samsa, G., Tierney, W., Belyea, M. and Hiner, S. (1992) Generic versus disease specific health status measures: comparing the Sickness Impact Profile and the Arthritis Impact Measurement Scales, *Journal of Rheumatology* 19: 543–6.

Weisman, M.H. (1989) Natural history and treatment decisions in rheumatoid arthritis revisited, *Arthritis Care and Research* 2 (3): S75–83.

Weisman, C.S. and Teitelbaum, M.A. (1985) Physician gender and the physician–patient relationship: recent evidence and relevant questions, *Social Science and Medicine* 10: 1119–27.

Weiss, R.S. (1976) The provisions of social relationships, in Z. Rubin (ed.), *Doing Unto Others*, Englewood Cliffs, NJ: Prentice Hall, pp. 17–26.

Wells, K., Stewart, A., Hays, R., Burnham, A., Rogers, W., Daniels, M., Berry, S., Greenfield, S. and Ware, J. (1989) The functioning and well-being of depressed patients, *Journal of American Medical Association* 262: 914–19.

Wenger, N. (1990) Gender, coronary artery disease, and coronary bypass surgery, *Annals of Internal Medicine* 112: 557–8.

West, C. (1993) Reconceptualizing gender in physician–patient relationships, *Social Science and Medicine* 36: 57–66.

Whitney, C.W. and von Korff, M. (1992) Regression to the mean in treated vs untreated pain?, *Pain* 50: 281–5.

Wiener, C. (1975) The burden of rheumatoid arthritis: tolerating the uncertainty, *Social Science and Medicine* 9: 97–104.

Williams, G.H. (1984) The genesis of chronic illness: narrative reconstruction, *Sociology of Health and Illness* 6: 175–200.

— (1986) Lay beliefs about the causes of rheumatoid arthritis: their implications for rehabilitation, *International Rehabilitation Medicine* 8: 65–8.

— (1987) Disablement and the social context of daily activity, *International Disability Studies* 9: 97–102.

— (1989) Hope for the humblest? The role of self-help in chronic illness: the case of ankylosing spondylitis, *Sociology of Health and Illness* 11: 135–59.

— (1993) Chronic illness and the pursuit of virtue in everyday life, in A. Radley (ed.), *Worlds of illness: biographical and cultural perspectives on health and disease,* London: Routledge.

Williams, G.H., Rigby, A.S. and Papageorgiou, A.C. (1992) Back to front? Examining research priorities in rheumatology, *British Journal of Rheumatology* 31: 193–6.

Williams, G.H. and Wood, P.H.N (1986) Common-sense beliefs about illness: a mediating role for the doctor, *Lancet* II: 1435–7.

— (1988) Coming to terms with chronic illness: the negotiation of autonomy in rheumatoid arthritis, *International Disability Studies* 10: 128–32.

Wills, T.A. (1985) Supportive functions of interpersonal relationships, in S. Cohen and S.L. Syme (eds), *Social support and health*, New York: Academic Press, pp. 61–82.

Wilske, K.R. and Healy, L.A. (1989) Remodeling the pyramid: a concept whose time has come, *Journal of Rheumatology* 16: 565–7.

Wolfe, F. and Cathey, M. (1991) The assessment and prediction of functional disability in rheumatoid arthritis, *Journal of Rheumatology* 18: 1298–1306.

Wolfe, F., Hawley, D. and Cathey, M. (1991) Clinical and health status measures over time: prognosis and outcome assessment in rheumatoid arthritis, *Journal of Rheumatology* 18: 1290–7.

Wolfe, R., Hawley, D. and Latham, M. (1990) Termination of slow acting antirheumatic therapy in rheumatoid arthritis: a 14 year prospective evaluation of 1017 consecutive starts, *Journal of Rheumatology* 17: 994–1002.

Wolfe, F. and Pincus, T. (1991) Standard self-report questionnaires in routine clinical research practice – an opportunity for patients and rheumatologists, *Journal of Rheumatology* 18: 643–6.

Wood, P.H.N. and Badley, E. (1986) Epidemiology of individual rheumatic disorders, in J.T. Scott (ed.), *Copeman's textbook of the rheumatic diseases*, sixth edition, London: Churchill Livingstone, pp. 59–142.

World Health Organization (1980) *International classification of impairments, disabilities, and handicaps*, Geneva: WHO.

Wortman, C.B. and Conway, T.L. (1985) The role of social support in adaptation and recovery from physical illness, in S. Cohen and S.L. Syme (eds), *Social support and health*, New York: Academic Press, pp. 281–302.

Wright, V. and Hopkins, R. (1977) Communicating with the rheumatic patient, *Rheumatology and Rehabilitation* 16: 107–18.

Yelin, E., (1992) The cumulative impact of a common chronic condition, *Arthritis and Rheumatism* 35(5): 489–97.

Yelin, E., Henke, C. and Epstein, W. (1987) The work dynamics of the person with rheumatoid arthritis, *Arthritis and Rheumatism* 30 (5): 507–12.

Yelin, E.H., Henke, C.J. and Epstein, W.V. (1986) Work disability among persons with musculoskeletal conditions, *Arthritis and Rheumatism* 29: 1322–33.

Yelin, E., Meenan, R., Nevitt, M., *et al.* (1980) Work disability in rheumatoid arthritis, *Annals of Internal Medicine* 93: 551–6.

Yelin, E., Nevitt, M., and Epstein, W. (1980) Toward an epidemiology of work disability, *Millbank Memorial Fund Quarterly/Health and Society* 58 (3): 386–415.

Young, L.D. (1992) Psychological factors in rheumatoid arthritis, *Journal of Consulting and Clinical Psychology* 60 (4): 619–27.

Zaphiropoulos, G. and Burry, H.C. (1974) Depression in rheumatoid disease, *Annals of the Rheumatic Diseases* 33: 132.

Zautra, A. and Manne, S.L. (1992) Coping with rheumatoid arthritis: a review of a decade of research, *Annals of Behavioral Medicine* 14(1): 31–9.

Ziebland, S., Fitzpatrick, R. and Jenkinson, C. (1993) Tacit models of disability underlying health status instruments, *Social Science and Medicine* 37: 69–75.

Ziebland, S., Fitzpatrick, R., Jenkinson, C., Mowat, A. and Mowat, A. (1992) Comparison of two approaches to measuring change in health status in rheumatoid arthritis: the Health Assessment Questionnaire (HAQ) and modified HAQ, *Annals of Rheumatic Diseases* 51: 1202–5.

Index